Natural Cures:

200 All Natural Fruit & Veggie Remedies

for Weight Loss, Health and Beauty

Gina 'The Veggie Goddess' Matthews

Copyright

DEDICATION

This book is dedicated to all those who recognize, appreciate and embrace all the natural remedies that our gifted to us, through the generosity of Mother Nature and the Divine Universe.

TABLE OF CONTENTS

Disclaimer:

The contents of this book are intended to be for educational, informational and entertainment purposes only. None of the information contained within this book writing is meant to be a substitute for professional medical advice, and the author and publisher recommend that you be under the care and guidance of a qualified health practitioner. If you currently take medication for any health condition, do not stop or alter your medication without first consulting your doctor. The author and publisher are not responsible for any use, or misuse, of any information contained within this book.

INTRODUCTION

I think all of us have been exposed to natural remedies at one time or another in our lives, and I truly feel we are returning, to this more natural way of living. Natural healing and the use of natural remedies, is not meant to shun modern medicine. Instead, it is a safe and oftentimes harmless first defense, against life's constant barrage of both minor and major threats to our health and well-being.

The promise of modern medicine, actually of the pharmaceutical industry, was that there would be a drug available for every disease. They've certainly kept to that promise, and there is no question, that there have been some miraculous pharmaceutical discoveries. Unfortunately, it has also led to the corruption and misuse of pharmaceuticals, and the public is all-to-aware of all the harsh side effects and consequences, long-term use of pharmaceutical drugs can bring. The drug manufacturers are never content with their inventory of drugs they already have for every major ailment. They are constantly creating new drugs for the prevention of diseases, however minute and unlikely, and pushing them onto the public irresponsibly. Drug trial results are commonly misrepresented, and instead of educating the public on prevention, via natural nutrition and lifestyle, the drug companies mode of operation, is to instead fill your head with the thought that there is a pill you can take for anything your heart desires, consequences be damned. And, the drug manufacturers, with the help from not-so-ethical lobbyists, will often warn the public against the 'dangers' of using natural remedies. It doesn't take a genius to figure out why that is. Keeping those high profits rolling in is serious business.

Using natural remedies is not meant to discourage your use of pharmaceutical drugs, in the event that you truly do need them. Instead, natural remedies are encouraged to be used as a means of preventative health measure, as well as a means of less caustic and effective ways to reverse both internal and external health imbalances. Additionally, using natural remedies in adjunct with pharmaceuticals can help prevent your body from experiencing the many side effects that often occur when using pharmaceutical drugs.

Using natural foods both internally and externally is how our bodies were meant to survive and thrive. Our bodies naturally know how to assimilate nutrients and medicinal compounds found in foods, vs. synthetically manufactured ones, and unlike their lab-made counterparts, natural remedies have far less incidence of side effects. Typically, any side effects realized when using natural remedies, is a result of a food allergy, or irresponsible use by the end user. And, just as is the case with pharmaceutical drugs, more is not better, and you always want to use what is known as MED, or minimum effective dose.

With all the foods listed in the book, it is always highly recommended that you use organic options as much as you possibly can. I can't overstate enough how dangerous the constant accumulation of chemical herbicides and insecticides is to both your mental and physical body. These chemical residues can never be completely washed off, no matter how good or natural the produce wash solution is. And, the majority of these chemical residues tend to stay saturated in the peels and rinds of both fruits and vegetables. So, if you can't find or afford organic produce, at least always remove and discard the outer peels and rinds from non-organic, commercial produce.

And, for remedy recipes that include honey, always only use raw honey. Not 'natural', or 'pure' honey, but 100% raw honey only. Raw honey is unfiltered, unpasteurized and unadulterated in any way, leaving all the nutrients and live enzymes intact. All other types of honey have been processed in some way, and as a result of this processing, it destroys the nutrients and live enzymes that give honey its medicinal value. In fact, recent studies have exposed that almost 80% of commercial honey sold in stores, is actually a processed mixture of honey and corn syrup, displaying another sad example of the corruption found in the commercial food industry, and that is not corrected by the so-called consumer advocate group, the FDA.

And finally, please realize that while natural remedies are highly effective, one size does not fit all. Every one of us is a unique human being, with very unique metabolic nuances. These unique metabolic nuances are constantly changing, and are the combined results of our diet, any past or present injuries, illnesses or disease, past and present drug and supplement use, and of course, genetic factors. In other words, no one natural remedy will yield the same result for every single person who uses it. One person may find grand success at dissolving warts from one particular remedy, while another may have to do a little bit of trial and error to find the natural wart remedy that works best for them.

Please also always take into consideration any possible food allergies that you may have, and do not use remedies that call for a particular food that you have (or may have) an allergy to. The same warning applies to those who have certain health conditions that would be further aggravated by the consumption of certain foods, as would be the case of someone with diverticulitis. These persons would not want to consume any natural remedies with foods that contained tiny seeds, such as are found in strawberries. In cases where the natural remedy calls for external use, then the same precautions may not be necessary. Just always use good judgment, and always be sure to discuss any questions that you may have about natural remedies, with a qualified health practitioner.

So, without further ado, let's explore some of the wonderful natural remedies Mother Nature has to offer us for weight loss, health and beauty.

Bon Veggie Appetit!

Gina 'The Veggie Goddess' Matthews

Apples:

Apples are not only a favorite fruit amongst the vast variety of fruit available, they are also one of nature's tried and true whole body detoxifiers. Keeping the body cleansed of toxins, pollutants, chemicals and pathogens, is crucial for effortlessly maintaining a healthy weight, keeping illness and disease away, and helping your skin to stay smooth and youthful looking. The unique thing about the shelf life of harvested apples is that even minor imperfections (cuts, tears, bruises, wrinkling) will speed deterioration, yet with proper storage, an un-marred apple can last a long time. The very best way to store apples is to gently wrap them individually in newspaper, and stack them loosely in a crate or bin in a cool, dark location. Apples will perish in freezing temperatures, as well as temperatures that are too high, so avoid storing in the garage. If you take the time to store apples this way, you can take advantage of a large harvest or purchase, and your apples should stay fresh for 1-2 months.

1. Apples are powerful infection fighters, and contain some penicillin-like properties. Eating a fresh, organic apple 3 times a day can knock out a stomach-flu, cold and other common viruses quick, having you back on your feet in no time. If it is a flu you are

suffering from, then consuming nothing but organic apples and water and tea will help to quickly neutralize and flush pathogens from your body, while supplying your body with much needed nutrients. This is a much better alternative to consuming soda pop and crackers.

2. Apples are very effective for remedying acute diarrhea, or 'Montezuma's Revenge', which is often a common malady when traveling to other countries. Take 1-2 large, ripe apples (preferably organic) and grate it, allowing the pulp to stand at room temperature for several hours until considerably darkened before eating. The grated fruit develops oxidized pectin, and is the same base ingredient used in the popular pink anti-diarrhea medicine you find over-the-counter. It is important for you to let the grated apple turn completely brown before eating, otherwise you will not get these same benefits.

3. To effortlessly reduce your caloric intake, shed excess pounds and maintain a healthy weight set-point, eat an organic apple 15-30 minutes before every meal. This works better than any so-called magic diet pill that seems to come out on the market on an almost weekly basis. The natural dietary fiber contained in apples will help slow the digestive process, which means you'll feel fuller sooner and stay fuller longer. Apples

also have a high water content, and food high in water content not only fill us up faster, but they satisfy our hunger and prevent overeating and unhealthy food cravings.

4. If you suffer from any type of digestive disorder, such as constipation, irritable bowel syndrome, heartburn, excess gas, etc., eating an apple prior to meals can greatly help to alleviate your symptoms. Apples help to stimulate the flow of digestive juices which are necessary for the proper assimilation of the food and beverage you take in, while at the same time neutralizing harmful stomach and intestinal bacteria, making for a much healthier and effective remedy vs. over-the-counter indigestion and heartburn medications (which by the way, are designed to ONLY be taken for a maximum of 2 weeks, otherwise they will bring upon 'rebound symptoms').

5. You can also use apples in the form of apple cider vinegar. Never ingest white vinegar. You only want to use organic apple cider vinegar that contains the 'mother', which is the active, live enzymes contained within the vinegar. My personal favorite brand, which is extremely reputable, is Braggs brand apple cider vinegar. Just a sampling of the extraordinary number of uses of apple cider vinegar include: Neutralizing a sunburn and healing damaged skin, when a

soaked gauze is applied to the affected areas. Instantly relieves the pain, swelling and itching of insect bites and stings. Removes dandruff when used as a hair rinse after shampooing hair. Eliminates body odor when used in place of underarm deodorant. Remedies painful athlete's feet, when feet are soaked daily in a 50/50 mixture of water and apple cider vinegar. This will actually also rid feet of offensive odors as well, and is incredibly effective if your feet are hot and sweaty after a long day's work.

Asparagus:

Asparagus is actually a member of the lily family, and comes in green, white and purple varieties. Asparagus needs to be cooked before consuming, and if you're diabetic and watching your sugar intake, you'll want to stay away from the purple variety, as it's much higher in sugar than the green and white variety of asparagus. And, if you've ever wondered why your urine smells funny after eating asparagus, it's due to the fact that once it's digested, it creates a sulfur-like compound, which is responsible for the strong urine odor you might notice as soon as 15 minutes after consuming. Asparagus deteriorates quickly after harvest, so it's imperative that you choose healthy specimens at the store or farmers market, and only purchase what you'll consume in 1-2 days. You want to select stalks that are firm and uniform in color (should be bright green) and texture. The ends of the stalks should never be limp or excessively dry. The best way to store asparagus if you're not going to use them right away is upright in a container with about ½ inch of water at the bottom, as asparagus requires lots of moisture.

1. Asparagus is a superior source of potassium and contains the amino acid asparagine. These two components combine for a powerful diuretic effect and cleansing of harmful acid waste within the body, bringing much sought after relief from gout, arthritis and rheumatism symptoms, such as pain, swelling and stiffness. Diuretics are also effective at breaking down fat deposits within the body, allowing for easier removal through our excretory system. In other words, it makes it easier for your body to flush out the nasty stuff. What many people don't know is that when our body retains water, it isn't 'just' water. Its water filled with toxic waste. And, if this toxic water buildup remains in our body for any extended amount of time, it will start to have detrimental effects on our joints, skin and organs. Drinking lots of filtered water and eating fresh asparagus will help keep your body from storing toxic fluid, thus preventing and relieving a lot of health

imbalances.

2. Did you know that asparagus is a powerful and highly effective hangover remedy? Asparagus is high in several amino acids that stimulate the enzyme functions necessary for the breakdown and removal of alcohol within the body. Eating asparagus before an evening filled with cocktails (or the morning after) helps to speed the body's metabolizing and detoxification process of alcohol, making for a shorter-lived episode of hangover symptoms, or preventing you from even feeling them in the first place. How much is enough? Eating 6 cooked asparagus spears, along with plenty of water before and after drinking will help do the trick.

3. Asparagus is a very beneficial vegetable to eat regularly, if you're trying to lose weight. It contains the chemical asparagine, an alkaloid that stimulates the kidneys and circulatory process. This particular alkaloid has a direct effect on the cells, and the breakdown of fat within the body. Asparagus helps to remove waste and fats from the body, by breaking up and dissolving the oxalic acid , an acid that 'glues' fat to body cells. Combine asparagus's diuretic abilities, with this detoxification process, and you have a very powerful and safe weight loss effect.

4. Looking to slow down the effects of aging, and strengthen your bones? In addition to containing calcium, magnesium, protein, vitamin A, vitamin C, vitamin E, riboflavin, thiamin, iron, copper, niacin and phosphorus, asparagus is the top source of vitamin K, the main nutrient in the development and maintenance of bone density. Eating asparagus regularly will help aid cardiac dysfunctions, due to its high phosphorus content, and its diuretic effect of eliminating potentially dangerous excess water in the body, especially surrounding the heart. Asparagus also contains the ever-vital antioxidant, glutathione, which helps combat cellular inflammation and is scientifically proven to slow down the aging process within the body.

5. Ladies, if you're looking to reduce the appearance of unwanted cellulite on your hips and thighs, be sure to add lots of asparagus into your diet. Asparagus flushes toxins from the body, strengthens veins and capillaries, and is loaded with collagen building nutrients that are needed to smooth the unsightly dimpled appearance of cellulite. Removing trapped toxins, and strengthening your body's circulatory system is crucial, if you desire smooth, sexy skin. Because we've become a very sedentary society, sitting on our tushes for extended periods of time every day, it's easy for toxins and waste fluids to become

trapped in the cell tissues of our buttocks and legs. Regular, moderate exercise (especially walking and swimming), along with ½-1 cup of steamed asparagus daily can help do wonderful things to change the appearance of your cellulite, transforming your legs from bumpy to bodacious.

Avocados:

Avocados are a fruit, with an absolutely amazing range of health benefits. It grows readily in the Mediterranean, Mexico and South American regions, and the majority of avocados grown in the United States come from California. Avocados supply the body with healthy fats that the body requires for weight loss, good skin health and optimal functions of all the systems within the human body. Unripe avocados take about 3-5 days to ripen at room temperature, and should be kept out of direct sunlight. Once ripened, you want to use them within 1-2 days. If you only need to use half of an avocado, you can keep it fresh by drizzling a squeeze of fresh lemon or lime juice across it to prevent oxidation, wrap it tightly in plastic wrap (not aluminum foil), and store in the fridge. If your avocados are already ripe when your purchase them, then it's best to store them in the fridge and use them within a few days. Color is not always an indicator of ripeness, because of the different avocado varieties. Therefore, a touch test is the best way to measure ripeness. Place the avocado in the palm of your hand, and give it a gentle squeeze (not too hard). If it feels hard and has no give, it is not yet ripe. If it gives just a bit when squeezed, it is ripe. If it is quite soft, it is past ripeness and should not be purchased.

1. If you want to keep your skin looking young, taut and fresh, doing a once-a-week avocado facial will produce results your friends will definitely take notice to. Just mash a fully ripe avocado, and you can either apply it to freshly washed skin 'as-is', or add a touch of raw honey (for mature, dry or sun-damaged skin), a touch of pure aloe (for sensitive skin, rosacea, eczema and psoriasis sufferers), or a pinch of bentonite clay (for acnes and oily skin). Apply liberally to face and neck area, and leave on for 15-30 minutes. Rinse with cool water and apply a mineral-free moisturizer.

2. The bulk of avocados calories are from its fat content, but don't let that scare you, because it's the healthy fat your body requires. And, when you feed your body healthy fats, instead of trans-fats, it signals the body to release the stored fat within your body's tissues. In other words, your body needs fat, to lose fat. It's a matter of giving your body the RIGHT kind of fat that is

crucial for losing excess weight and cellulite stores. What's the magic amount to eat for successful weight loss? 1-2 whole avocados a day. Just make sure to not eat them with a bag of chips, otherwise you'll offset the benefits. Cut them up and add them to your salad and vegetable dishes. Mash them, and use as a healthy sandwich spread with a sprinkle of real sea salt. You'll quickly notice your hunger pangs and food cravings will also disappear, which is another result of feeding your body healthy fats and nutrients.

3. If you struggle with constipation issues, try this healthy avocado digestive remedy that can bring you quick relief without any of those unwanted side effects from drugs and over-the-counter medications. First, you want to drink a full glass of cold water 15-30 minutes before consuming the avocado mash, to stimulate your digestive tract. Then, mash up 1-2 ripe avocados in a bowl, add in ½ tablespoon apple cider vinegar and ½ tablespoon of fresh squeezed lemon juice. You can sprinkle in some sea salt if you need to for taste. Eat the mash 'as-is', or spread it on a piece of sprouted whole grain bread (do not spread it on regular white or wheat bread, you need the REAL thing). This typically will stimulate a healthy bowel movement within 1-4 hours.

4. Avocados can also do wonders if you're

looking to stimulate hair growth, as well as improve the condition of your hair. Avocado are rich in oleic acids and omega-6 essential fatty acids, both vital for stimulating hair growth, and protecting the hair shaft against damage from hot hair appliances, hair coloring, wind, sun, cold and other harsh weather elements. To make an avocado hair mask, first gently brush out any hair product residue with a brush. Mash a large, ripe avocado in a bowl, and add in ½ cup olive oil OR coconut oil and whisk together until well blended. Apply the avocado mask to your hair from the scalp all the way to the ends, gently massaging your scalp as you are applying. If you have longer hair, double this recipe, and if you have short hair, you can cut the recipe in half. Once fully worked through your hair, and all strands are nicely saturated, cover your hair with a shower cap, and let sit for at least 1 hour, or longer if you can. Rinse out the avocado from your hair in the shower with cool water, shampoo twice, then condition. To stimulate new hair growth, massage your scalp with the pads of your fingers through the shower cap. If you have excessively oily hair, omit the oil from this recipe, and substitute with plain yogurt.

5. Avocados are a great nutritional prevention against heart issues, stroke and high cholesterol. Avocados are extremely rich in folate, a nutrient proven to help reduce the incident of heart dysfunctions, stroke and

even age-related eye disorders. And, numerous studies have found that eating an avocado a day, along with a healthy diet, was able to help study participants lower their bad cholesterol levels by up to 17% in just 1 week! Avocados are the top fruit source for vitamin E, as well as glutathione, a powerhouse antioxidant responsible for preventing aging, cancer and heart disease.

Bananas:

It might surprise you to know, that the majority of common bananas are actually genetically the same, because they come from trees that have been cloned for decades. 1950's to be exact. A banana is richer in antioxidants once it becomes ripe, giving it a slightly higher nutritional value over un-ripened bananas. If you're diabetic, or just plain watching your sugar intake, as a banana ripens from green to yellow, the starch is converted to sugar, so it will affect your blood glucose levels quicker. When you eat a banana when it's still green, your body must first breakdown and covert the starch content, which means a slower rise in blood glucose levels vs. eating a ripe banana, so choose which option is best for you.

1. Warts are said to not be able to tolerate

exposure to potassium. Perhaps this is why banana peels are so highly effective at quickly getting rid of them. Wherever you have a wart (hands, feet, etc.) cut a piece of banana peel large enough to fully cover the wart area, and using medical tape, tape the banana peel to the area, making sure to place the inside white pithy part of the peel against your skin. You can store the remaining peel in a plastic baggie in the fridge, and cut up piece as you need them. For best results, replace the peel twice a day, and within a week you should start noticing your wart(s) shrinking and disappearing away. For stubborn warts, swab the affected area with apple cider vinegar and allow to air dry before wrapping with the banana peel.

2. Bananas are surprisingly good for bone health. Too many people's diets are high in sodium, which leaches calcium from bones and expels it out with your urine. Bananas high potassium content, are responsible for helping to prevent calcium loss. In addition, bananas are also rich in fructooligosaccharide (FOS), that along with insulin, help the body to uptake and efficiently absorb calcium. This chemical reaction helps strengthen bone density and reduce the risk of osteoporosis as we age.

3. If you're concerned about good digestive health, bananas are brimming with benefits to help ease and prevent many digestive

complaints. Eating bananas triggers the production of a stomach protecting mucus, providing a natural buffer against stomach acid, which helps to reduce and even prevent painful stomach ulcers. Bananas secondary protection against stomach ulcers is due to its protease inhibitors, which breakdown harmful bacteria that might otherwise contribute to a stomach ulcer. Bananas can also bring relief for both constipation and diarrhea. Bananas pectin content helps to get things moving in the digestive tract, thereby helping to relieve constipation. On the flip-side, bananas high potassium content can help to bring the digestive system back into balance, during a bout of diarrhea. Potassium is one of the main minerals (electrolytes) lost during bouts of diarrhea and vomiting, and needs to be replaced.

4. Rubbing the inside of a ripe banana peel against your skin can bring about many a skin beautifying remedy. If you suffer from psoriasis, liberally rubbing the inside of a banana peel across your affected areas twice a day, will bring rapid relief to your itching, swelling and redness within just a few days. Same goes for when you get an insect or bug bite. As soon as you can, rub the bite area with the inside of the peel, to help reduce the itching, swelling and inflammation caused by the toxins release into your skin from the offending insect or bug. And, to help reduce acne breakouts, after you wash your face

with a gently soap and remove any traces of makeup and dirt, generously rub the inside of a banana peel across your entire face. You should start to notice a lessening of your acne symptoms within a few days to a week. In all cases, once you rub the inside of the peel against your skin, allow your skin to air dry, and you can wash off any residual residue later, or the next morning with cool water.

5. While many people think bananas are fattening, you'd be surprised to learn they are proving to be quite the healthy weight loss aid. Un-ripened bananas (peel is mostly green) contain a very high content of a substance known as 'resistant starch'. This resistant starch does magical things to your metabolism, by helping to preserve muscle, making you feel fuller longer (thereby squashing hunger pains and cravings), and as it passes through your system (vs. being stored and deposited as fat), it actually helps to shrink fat cells. To get the most of these weight loss benefits, eat 2 un-ripened bananas each morning for breakfast, along with water, herbal tea or black coffee. Studies have shown that eating resistant starch in the morning vs. at other times during the day has a heightened ability to prevent dieters from over-eating throughout the course of the day.

Berries:

Within the wonderful world of fruits, berries rank right at the top, when it comes to antioxidant content. Antioxidants are necessary in one's diet, to neutralize and eliminate harmful free radicals within the body. Antioxidants help fend off the ravages of age-related health conditions, as well as help to keep wrinkles away and skin looking bright, clear and youthful. Eating nothing but fresh berries when you are sick will help to quickly flush pathogens from your body, while supporting your health and hastening your recovery, due to their amazing antioxidant and nutrient content. When purchasing berries, you want to choose ones that you can either hand-pick from a bulk bin at your farmers market, or in a shallow, ventilated plastic crate or container. Berries keep fresh when stored on a middle shelf of your fridge, stored towards the back, and kept in its original container. If you've purchased them from a bulk bin at a farmers market, then place them in a brown paper bag with the end left open for ventilation. Depending on their ripeness when purchased, berries will stay fresh for 3-7 days after purchase and proper storage.

1. Whether you suffer from the occasional pimple breakout, or have been battling acne forever, strawberries are a natural way to help combat those breakouts. Strawberries

are a naturally rich source of salicylic acid, the main ingredient used in many over-the-counter and prescription acne medications. To use, gently mash up a few ripe strawberries, and apply as a mask after first washing skin with a mild non-soap facial cleanser. Let sit for 30 minutes then rinse with cool water. Allow face to air dry. In addition to helping dry out and eliminate those unwanted pimples, the fresh strawberry mash will also help to brighten skin tone, tighten your pores, and even help to lighten and fade scars and other skin discolorations.

2. While most women are aware that consuming cranberries can help prevent and relieve urinary tract infections (UTI's), you may not know that blueberries are also quite effective at keeping the bladder tract clear of infection-causing bacteria. Firstly, blueberries high antioxidant content, help the body to fend off bacterial infections. Secondly, blueberries are rich in a substance called 'arbutin compounds', which not only have natural antibiotic properties, but they are also responsible for inhibiting harmful bacteria from latching onto the lining of the bladder, thereby keeping the bladder and urinary tract clean and free of bacterial colonization and infection.

3. If you're looking to solve a particular hair concern, such as premature graying of your

hair, excessive hair loss, or oily scalp, gooseberries are tried and true for helping to reverse these unwanted conditions. In a saucepan filled with about 1 cup of unrefined coconut oil (do not use refined coconut oil), toss in a handful of fresh gooseberries, and gently bring to a boil. Continue to cook until mixture has turned black. Remove from heat and allow to fully cool. Once cooled, keep in a sealed container at room temperature. Use this prepared oil 3 times a week as a scalp massage treatment. Massage the oil into your scalp using the pads of your fingers, for 10 minutes, then cover with a shower cap. Leave on for another hour, or overnight if you can. Be sure to protect your bedding by putting a large old towel across your pillow. Shampoo twice in the morning, to fully remove the gooseberry oil.

4. For those suffering from painful conditions such as arthritis, gout and rheumatism, cranberries have been proven to help bring amazing relief from your symptoms. All 3 of these conditions involve having too much uric acid within the body, especially the joint areas. This excess uric acid actually crystallizes around the joint areas, causing limited mobility, pain, stiffness and swelling. Cranberries help to reduce painful inflammation, aid in breaking-up and flushing out stored crystalline deposits, and help prevent future accumulation of uric

acid in the body. For starters, try replacing your daily coffee or black tea with fresh brewed cranberry tea instead. You can readily purchase cranberry tea at any health food store, and make a strong cup by steeping for 10 minutes before drinking. You can also drink some fresh cranberry juice, by combining 1 ounce of PURE cranberry concentrate with 8-10 ounces of filtered water, and aim for drinking 3 glasses a day. And, don't forget to try adding in some fresh chopped cranberries to your salads, oatmeal and even just as a snack throughout the day.

5. For certain skin conditions, blackberries are ideal for bringing about quick relief from skin rashes, acne, psoriasis, sun damage and aging skin. Credit goes to blackberries high acid and tannin content. To use, mash up a handful of fresh, ripe blackberries, and spread across affected skin areas. Allow to air dry and sit for at least 30-60 minutes, before rinsing with cool water.

6. A must-have natural remedy to keep in every household, for ready use in treating coughs, sore throats, inflamed tonsils, colds and flu's, is grandma's elderberry syrup. It's so easy to make, and lasts for up to 3 months in the fridge. To make, you need 1 full cup of fresh elderberries, 3 cups of water, and 1 cup of raw honey (do NOT use processed honey). Heat the elderberries and water in a

saucepan over medium heat, until mixture comes to a boil. Let mixture gently boil for 1 minute, then reduce heat and simmer for 30 minutes. Remove from heat and mash up the berries using a fork or potato masher. Strain mixture through a mesh strainer into a bowl, and whisk in the raw honey until well blended. Once cooled, transfer into a glass mason jar (or something similar that can be tightly sealed), and store in the fridge. Will keep for up to 3 months. When needed, suggested dose is 1 teaspoon every 2-3 hours. Do not give to children under the age of 2 years, due to the honey content.

7. For a once a week natural teeth whitening treatment, here's another great home use for strawberries. Slice a large, ripe strawberry in half and rub the cut-sides of the strawberry across the surface of all your teeth. Let residue sit on your teeth for 5 minutes, then dip a moistened toothbrush into some plain baking soda, and brush your teeth for 1-2 full minutes. Rinse thoroughly with water, and wait 30 minutes before eating or drinking anything. While this is a very effective natural teeth whitening remedy, all good things in moderation, so do not use more than once a week.

8. To keep your face looking fresh, smooth and wrinkle-free, try this amazing anti-aging blueberry facial mask. Mash together equal parts of fresh blueberries with plain yogurt.

Apply to freshly washed skin, and allow mixture to sit on skin for 30-60 minutes. The natural fruit acids in the blueberries and the lactic acid in the yogurt will gently exfoliate dead skin, while at the same time naturally stimulating your skin's collagen production. Lack of collagen is what makes our skin thin, droop, sag and form wrinkles. As we age, our skin also doesn't shed its' deaden layers as readily, resulting in ashen, dull looking skin. Natural and gentle exfoliation is important in ridding the skin of accumulated dead skin cells and keeping the skin bright and taught.

9. If you are looking to speed up your weight loss efforts in a natural and healthy way, then be sure to incorporate 1-2 cups of fresh strawberries, blueberries or raspberries into your daily diet. Not only are they low in calories, but they contain natural plant fibers to help keep your digestive system moving. Berries are brimming with fat-fighting antioxidants, which are necessary in preventing cellular inflammation and fat storage within the body, and they are also all natural appetite suppressants. Eating ½ cup of fresh berries 30 minutes before a meal is proven to reduce your caloric intake at that meal, as well as prevent cravings for unhealthy food choices throughout the rest of the day.

10. Juniper berries are an often overlooked berry

and an unsung hero when it comes to alleviating a host of digestive complaints. Juniper berries are a natural digestive aid, and a main ingredient used in 'bitters' tonic, to relieve indigestion, heartburn and excess gas. They have also been successfully used to stimulate urine flow and the dissolving of kidney stones and gallstones. Juniper berries impart powerful cleansing and detoxification properties to the kidneys, bladder and prostate. Juniper berries have a rather bitter taste when eating alone, so they are best enjoyed when mixed into a smoothie, fruit sauce or marinade.

Cabbage:

Cabbage falls into the cruciferous vegetable category, and is one particular veggie you want to consume on a regular basis. Not only is cabbage a rich plant source of vitamin C, it is also abundant in vitamin K, folate, fiber, manganese, calcium, potassium and B6 vitamin. It can be eaten raw, juiced, steamed or cooked. You'll want to avoid buying a pre-cut head of cabbage, because while they are rich in vitamin C and other nutrients, once the cabbage is cut, their nutrient content quickly degrades. So, buy your cabbage whole and use it within a day or two after cutting. When storing cabbage, keep it tightly wrapped in plastic and place it in a crisper drawer in the fridge.

1. Taking antacids long-term (longer than 2 weeks), can have detrimental health effects. If you suffer from stomach ulcers, acid reflux and heartburn, you'll be happy to learn that multiple medical journals have confirmed the beneficial powers of raw cabbage and raw cabbage juice, in relieving and healing any kind of gastrointestinal ulcer, be it duodenal, peptic, etc.. Drinking ½ cup of raw cabbage juice twice daily (once in the morning, and once at night) is a natural antacid, plus a great ulcer healer, thereby reducing and even potentially eliminating heartburn, acid reflux and other symptoms.

2. If you have a wound, burn or skin condition, regular raw cabbage juice compresses will bring speedy relief from pain, and hasten healing. To make a compress, run a head of cabbage through a juicer, and soak a cheesecloth or handkerchief in the juice, wringing out any excess juice back into the bowl. Cover affected skin area (wound, burn, acne, eczema, psoriasis, rash) with the cabbage juice compress, followed by a layer of plastic wrap, to prevent drying out. Keep in place for 4 hours, remove, then allow air dry without rinsing. The high sulfur content in cabbage contains natural antibacterial,

antifungal and antiseptic properties, helping to quickly rid unwanted skin conditions and stimulate the rejuvenation and mending of healthy skin tissue and reducing the incidence of scarring. If you don't have a juicer, boil a head of cabbage until leaves are soft, and use the cooled liquid to make your compress. And, don't forget to add those freshly boiled cabbage leaves into your favorite veggie casserole or other vegetarian dish.

3. For pain relief from a pulled or strained muscle, menstrual cramps, arthritis, and so forth, you might find this particular remedy bizarre, yet surprisingly effective. Carefully tear a handful of large cabbage leaves from the cabbage head, and arrange in a single layer onto an ironing board. Cover with a thin towel, and setting your clothes iron to medium heat, carefully iron the cabbage leaves until they become velvety soft. (be sure to move iron constantly) Once the cabbage leaves are ironed to the correct texture, rub a thin layer of olive oil onto one side of each leaf, and place the leaves oiled-side down against the pain affected areas of your body. Cover with a heavy towel, heating pad or hot water bottle, and keep in place for 30 minutes or longer before removing. As bizarre as this this remedy sounds, the compounds in the cabbage leaves will quickly soothe away pain-inducing inflammation from the area,

bringing you quick relief from pain, swelling and stiffness.

4. Another great use for raw cabbage juice (or the boiled water from boiling cabbage), is to use it as a mouth wash and gargle when you have a sore throat, laryngitis, or mouth sores due to the herpes virus or as a result of chemotherapy. After brushing teeth, gargle with some cabbage juice for a full 1 minute before spitting out juice. Do NOT drink the gargled juice, for it will be infused with the pathogens it picked-up inside your mouth. Gargle every 4 hours until you find relief. You can also gargle daily as a preventative measure against mouth sores.

5. For frequent dieters, many of you have heard the wonders of a cabbage soup diet to lose excess weight fast. There are pros and cons of doing this, and the cons are mostly in the form of not following the recommended guidelines of this diet. Cabbage is a great weight loss-supporting vegetable, and you don't necessarily need to eat it in soup form to achieve healthy and permanent loss of fat, cellulite and pounds. Eating 5 servings of cabbage daily can help take the boredom out of a soup only protocol, while still allowing you to lose weight. It also means that you'll be eating other healthy foods along with the cabbage, along with 8-10 glasses of filtered water, so you're less likely to stray and food binge, as

you otherwise might due to the strictness of a soup and water only diet for 7 days. One of the ways cabbage aids in weight loss, is by stimulating the release of stored waste in the colon and digestive tract. In fact, for every 1 gram of cabbage you consume, your stool output will increase by up to 18 percent. This is a very healthy way to cleanse the colon, without using any harsh and habit-forming laxatives and other products. And, one of the first places you'll notice your weight loss, is around your midsection.

Carrots:

The ever-popular carrot is from the root vegetable family, and can typically be found on veggie trays at a party or gathering. Carrots are known for their ability to support eye health, but they actually possess a whole lot more health and beauty benefits than you might expect. In fact, a surprising hiccup remedy involves inhaling freshly grated carrots for 30-60 seconds, for quick relief of spasms. When purchasing carrots, always remove the green tops before storing, otherwise they'll pull moisture and nutrients away from the carrots after harvest. If stored away from other fruits and vegetables, and kept in their own crisper drawer in the fridge, carrots can keep for a lengthy 2-3 months. To get this amount of storage time from carrots, choose bright, firm, thick specimens, and keep stored in a tightly sealed plastic bag to retain moisture.

1. For an easy, yet highly effective anti-aging facial treatment, try this simple carrot mask. Boil 2-3 large carrots until soft. Mash cooked carrots thoroughly in a bowl, and stir in 2 tablespoons of raw honey (never eat or apply processed honey to skin). Once mixture is well blended, apply in an even layer to freshly washed skin, across face, neck and décolletage area. Let mixture stand for 30 minutes or more, before rinsing with cool water and applying a mineral oil-free moisturizer. Carrot's rich vitamin A and beta-carotene content, keep the effects of aging at bay, reducing and preventing fine lines, wrinkles, sagging skin and 'turkey neck'. Your skin will also become tighter, brighter and plumper with regular once to twice a week treatments.

2. Carrots are probably the best vegetable choice for cleansing your liver, and aiding in the detoxification of toxic wastes from the body. Carrots stimulate and strengthen the gallbladder's and liver's ability to process and purge toxic waste from the body, and is especially useful in supporting those who are in the process of overcoming drug and alcohol addictions. Carrots also are a quick

remedy in relieving constipation and eradicating intestinal parasites. For intense detoxification and digestive support, drink ½ cup of fresh carrot juice daily, or, you can eat 2 large fresh carrots a day as a snack or in your dishes.

3. A surprising remedy to help one kick the smoking habit, is noshing on a fresh carrot stick every time one gets the urge to smoke. There are several factors that help make this an effective smoking remedy. Firstly, a carrot stick feels a bit like holding a cigarette, so it helps replace the psychological need/habit of holding onto a cigarette. Secondly, carrots are naturally sweet, which has a suppressing factor on one's urge to smoke, yet it doesn't sabotage your health the way replacing cigarettes with candy does. And, thirdly, noshing on carrot sticks gives you a physical activity replacement to smoking, which helps take your mind off of your craving, to focus on your current activity. This carrot remedy is actually used in prisons all across Europe to successfully help prisoners stop smoking.

4. Do carrots actually help one's vision? The answer is 'yes', but, only night vision can be improved by eating carrots. When levels of light sensitive molecules are low, due to a vitamin A deficiency, there will not be enough retinal to detect light at night. However, even if one does have low levels

of retinal, there is enough light during the daytime hours to produce vision. If you do actually suffer from nighttime blindness, or have trouble driving at night, eating a carrot a day can help supply you with the extra retinol-supporting vitamin A that you might need.

5. And, I can't overlook the old hippie remedy for teething babies. Instead of giving your baby or grandbaby a store-bought teething ring to chew on during their teething phases, try giving them a cold or slightly frozen carrot stick instead. The cold will of course soothe the swelling and pain of the babies gums, and the natural sweetness of the carrot will entice the baby to gnaw on it, helping to further ease any discomfort, strengthen their gums and gently breakthrough those first baby teeth. And, as with any toy or baby device, do not ever leave a baby or child unattended when giving them something to chew or play with.

Celery:

Did you know that celery's name comes from Latin and means 'quick acting' due to its medicinal properties. While you may think of plain celery as just a bland tasting, it's actually exploding with minerals and other vital nutrients, and is an important vegetable to consume on a regular basis. And, while celery is high in nutrients and medicinal value, it is almost completely devoid of calories, making it a perfect 'go-to' snack for dieters, and pairs easily with other healthy foods, such as almond butter and hummus. When purchasing celery, you always want to opt for organic, as celery ranks as one of the highest vegetables to retain toxic pesticides and herbicides that are applied during commercial farming. You can't wash these residues off, and will therefore be ingesting these toxic substances when you consume the celery, so go organic.

1. A tonic commonly used in China to ease the symptoms of anxiety and stress, is an elixir made up of equal amounts of raw celery juice and raw honey (as always, never use processed honey). The suggested dosage is 2-3 tablespoons, 3 times a day, evenly spaced during your awakened hours. The seeds and stalks of celery both contain a sedative compound called 'phthalide', which is responsible for its sedative and calming properties. An alternative tonic, is to juice equal parts of celery and carrot together, and drink 6-8 ounces of this juice daily to strengthened frayed nerves and keep you stay centered and calm.

2. Sprinkling celery seeds to your dishes, or chewing on some after a meal, work

wonders at relieving and preventing common digestive complaints such as excess gas, indigestion and acid reflux. Celery seeds can also help to calm a spastic colon, as well as increase your urine output. Celery is a great veggie to regularly consume, for the prevention of kidney and gallstones.

3. If you struggle with symptoms of low-thyroid, such as weight gain, fatigue, low libido, muscle and joint pain, hair loss, depression, etc., you'll be happy to know, that eating raw celery has been proven to help stimulate and support the functioning of both the thyroid and pituitary glands, helping to alleviate your symptoms and assist in bringing these glands back into balance. Celery supplies you with organic sodium, the kind that is required by your body for proper functioning of all your body systems, vs. the unhealthy table salt that is sold in stores today. Without organic sodium, our organs would fail and we would die. On the flip-side, consuming chemically processed table salt also causes your organs to fail, which can ultimately lead to death. So, be sure to give your body the organic sodium it needs through natural dietary sources.

4. When it comes to cleansing the body of unwanted substances, celery possesses some powerful detoxification abilities. For

starters, celery is rich in important nutrients and unique antioxidants, which neutralize the damaging effects of free radicals. Free radicals cause cellular inflammation, which then leads to a whole host of undesirable health problems, so eating foods that are rich in antioxidants is crucial for good health. Secondly, celery is a great source of dietary fiber, providing the roughage needed to effectively sweep the digestive tract and colon of accumulated wastes, so that it can be expelled from the body. And, thirdly, celery is a gentle and safe diuretic, which aids in the flushing of trapped toxic fluids that might be stored in body tissues, which are responsible for weight gain, cellulite and health imbalances.

5. An effective home remedy for those who are battling chronic acne outbreaks consists of drinking a unique celery juice recipe blend. Chronic acne is the result of inflammation of the hair follicles and sebaceous glands of the skin. The mechanism of why this happens is unknown. However, what is known is a natural remedy that has been proven to bring visible clearing results within 1-2 weeks. To make this juice, combine 2 stalks of finely chopped celery, 1 large diced tomato, 1 large diced pear and ½ of a large lemon (segments without the peel) into a blender or juicer, and drink 1 cup daily in the morning on an empty stomach.

Cherries:

Cherries are a favorite summer fruit for many, and there are many varieties to choose from. The two main cherry classifications are sweet and tart, and both are loaded with unique antioxidants and other nutrients that support good health and beauty. If you're watching your sugar intake, tart cherry varieties contain about 40% less sugar than their sweet variety counterparts, as well as about 20% less calories as well. Sweet cherry varieties include Bing, Lambert and Rainier, while some of the popular tart cherry varieties include Montmorency and Balaton. When storing freshly purchased cherries, you want to keep them in a plastic bag, and get them into the fridge as soon as you can. Cherries can lose more quality in one hour at room temperature, than a day in the fridge. Also, never wash cherries until right before you're ready to use them, as the excess moisture will seep into the stems and lead to splits or premature spoilage of the fruit.

1. For those suffering from the painful conditions of arthritis, gout and rheumatism, cherries can bring safe and natural relief from your symptoms as effectively as NSAIDS (non-steroidal anti-inflammatories, such as ibuprofen, aspirin and naproxen). Cherries, just like NSAID's, contain a sub-

class of flavonoids called 'anthocyanidins', which are proven to block pain. In addition to blocking pain, cherries also help to reduce levels of uric acid within the body, thereby reducing the body's overall acidity levels, which help to reduce and prevent the occurrence of painful symptoms in the first place. Suggested dietary dosage is 20-25 fresh tart cherries daily, but you can also get these benefits from drinking pure cherry juice (no added sugar or additional ingredients), canned cherries and even dried cherries, with effectiveness being in that order.

2. Having trouble sleeping? You might be surprised to learn, that cherries are a rich, natural dietary source of the sleep hormone melatonin. Often dubbed the 'natural nightcap', eating tart cherries can help offset the effects jet lag, insomnia and other sleep disturbances, naturally and without any unwanted side effects. Even a slight increase in one's melatonin levels is proven to help restore natural sleep rhythms, helping one to fall asleep faster, as well as stay asleep once you fall asleep. Melatonin found from food sources, enters the bloodstream and binds with sites in the brain, where it helps restore the body's levels of melatonin, and enhance the natural sleep process. Suggested dosage is ½ cup dried cherries, 1 cup fresh or frozen cherries, or 2 tablespoons of pure cherry juice concentrate.

3. Cherries are a super-food for clear skin and anti-aging benefits. The high levels of vitamin A and beta carotene found in cherries help prevent the breakdown of collagen, which would otherwise lead to wrinkles, sagging and crepey-looking skin. Additionally, the elagic acid (a unique antioxidant) found in cherries promotes healthy skin cell rejuvenation and skin purity, resulting in more youthful and radiant looking skin. Even more skin benefits can be gotten from cherries, due to their high astringent properties, which help to clear acne, rashes and various skin conditions caused by inflammation. In addition to eating fresh cherries, you can also apply some mashed fresh cherries or pure cherry concentrate to freshly washed skin, and allow to air dry on skin before rinsing with cool water. This will help to balance out skin tone, dry out acne, tighten pores and relieve excess oiliness.

4. Cherries aren't just good for anti-aging skin care they are also good at preventing age-related health issues such as heart attack and stroke. Cherries contain cyclooxegenase inhibitors (COX), which block the enzyme responsible for atherosclerosis, thereby helping to reduce plaque buildup on artery walls, and artery restrictions and blockages. In addition, cherries contain a powerful antioxidant flavonoid called 'anthocyanins', which is a key nutrient in protecting and

preventing inflammatory ailments such as heart attack, stroke, colon cancer and fibromyalgia.

5. Cherries, tart cherries in particular, are especially effective when it comes to weight management. Tart cherries are loaded with the amino acid tyrosine, which is converted to dopamine in the body. Low levels of dopamine are often caused by stress and poor diet, and result in symptoms such as low libido, lack of motivation and addictions and uncontrolled food cravings and food binges. Regularly eating tart cherries (15-20 a day) can help restore dopamine to more balanced levels, thereby helping to reduce food cravings, overeating and other unhealthy eating habits. Proper levels of dopamine will also help provide you with the motivation you need to maintain a routine of regular, moderate exercise, further helping you to lose excess weight and keep it off.

Citrus Fruits:

Citrus fruits are another popular sector in the fruit kingdom. Citrus fruits grow in the warm regions of the world, and nowadays, can be easily found at your local market year-round, thanks to the wonders of modern transportation. A little history fact:

British seamen acquired their now famous nickname 'limey's' in the 19th century, after limes were added to their daily rum rations to prevent scurvy. Citrus fruits include lemons, limes, grapefruits, oranges, tangerines, clementines and kumquats. When purchasing citrus fruits, you want to look for firm, heavy pieces, with brightly colored skins. Ideally, you want to purchase just enough citrus for what you'll use within the week, and store them at room temperature, away from direct sunlight. To extend the life of your citrus, you can also store them in the vegetable crisper drawers in your fridge, where they'll keep for 2-3 weeks.

1. Citrus fruits are incredibly versatile, when it comes to dental care. If you tend to suffer from bleeding gums after brushing your teeth, try this easy lemon remedy. Take a section of fresh lemon peel, and rub the inside, white pithy part across your gums after each brushing. You should notice a reduction or even complete elimination of gum bleeding within just a couple days. If you are suffering from a mild toothache, while you're waiting to get in to see your dentist, try this tried-and-true lime remedy from the tropics, where they don't often have access to a dentist. Soak a cotton ball or thin cloth in pure, fresh lime juice and apply directly over affected area. Pain should start to subside within just a few minutes. And, as a natural teeth whitener,

twice a week brush your teeth with a combination of equal parts of fresh grapefruit juice, lemon juice and lime juice. Not only does this help to naturally whiten your teeth, but it will also help reduce tartar build-up. Note: Never suck on a wedge of fresh citrus, as prolonged contact with citric acid can cause serious deterioration of your teeth's enamel.

2. A unique remedy for fast relief from a pounding headache or migraine is a hot lemon water footbath. When a headache or migraine comes on, as soon as you, squeeze up the fresh juice of 1-2 ripe lemons into a footbath with hot water. Make the water as hot as your feet can tolerate. While sitting, stick your feet into the hot lemon water, and you should start to feel relief within 5-10 minutes, but, try to keep your feet in longer if you can. The hot lemon water dilates and expands the blood vessels in your feet and legs, shunting the excess blood from your head, down to your feet, bringing you rapid relief.

3. If you live or vacation in an area where there are lots of mosquitoes and other biting insects, make sure to always have lots of fresh lemon on hand. As a natural insect repellent, mix together the juice of 2-3 large, ripe lemons with 2 cups of distilled water in a spray bottle, and spray liberally over exposed areas of your skin before headed

outside. If you've already been bitten up by mosquitoes, flies or other insects, rub some fresh squeezed lemon juice on the insect bite areas as soon as you can, to quickly reduce pain, swelling and itching within minutes.

4. If you suffer from candida (yeast infection), grapefruit can quickly stop it in its tracts, and help bring your body back into a healthier balance. Fresh grapefruit contains antifungal, antiviral and antibacterial properties, making it a potent warrior against yeast and other infectious invaders. Suggested dietary dosage for positive effects, is to eat 2 ripe, red-variety grapefruit daily, until symptoms subside. Thereafter, you can eat 1 every other day for maintenance.

5. A natural remedy dating back to the sixth century B.C. for digestive upset is tangerine tea. If you suffer from indigestion, excess gas and bloating after meals, instead of an after-dinner cocktail or unhealthy soda drink, try this easy-to-make tea instead. Peel a fresh tangerine and boil it in 2 cups of water for 5 minutes. Remove the peels and drink as a tea, preferably while it is hot. Tangerines stimulate digestive juices necessary for proper food assimilation, as well as help soothe and calm a spastic digestive tract.

6. Asians have long since used a lime

concoction, to stimulate and maintain healthy weight loss. If you're looking to lose excess weight and smooth out cellulite, try drinking the following recipe. Squeeze the juice from 1 large (or 2 medium) limes into a glass of warmed distilled water, and stir in 1 teaspoon of raw honey (never use processed honey). Drink this within 30 minutes of waking on an empty stomach, and wait another 30 minutes after drinking, before consuming any additional food or beverage. If you want an even tangier flavor, squeeze in some extra lime juice, or sprinkle in a dash of fresh ground black pepper into the drink, but do not add any additional honey. The Western culture has come up with a similar drink of lemon, cayenne and water, but this is the original weight loss elixir used for centuries in other countries.

7. When cold and flu season rolls around, make sure you keep this easy kumquat tea recipe around, for quick relief from cough, sore throat and chest congestion. Wash 12-14 kumquats, but do not peel. Slice in half, and squeeze most of the juice from each piece into a saucepan filled with 2 cups of water, then toss in the squeezed fruit pieces. Bring mixture to a boil, immediately remove from heat, and let steep for 5 minutes. Strain out the fruit skins and pour into a tea cup or mug. Drink while still hot. If you need to sweeten the tea, use only stevia or ½ teaspoon of raw honey. Kumquats have

expectorant properties, to help loosen and release chest congestion, thereby drying up any mucus in the lungs. It also soothes irritated throat tissues and calms irritating coughs.

8. If you're plagued with the lumps and bumps of unsightly cellulite, grapefruit has been used for hundreds of years, to successfully diminish its appearance. Grapefruit stimulates the lymph system to release trapped toxins from skin tissues, so that they can be expelled out the body. Grapefruit also possesses natural astringent properties, which help to tone and tighten the skin. Grapefruit combined with manual massage of the cellulite affected areas, will help tone, tighten and smooth out dimply skin, so you don't have to hide behind long skirts and pants. Suggested dosage for effected cellulite relief, is to consume 3 red grapefruit daily. You can either eat 1 before each meal, or juice them all together with 2 stalks of celery, and drink this as your morning meal. If you do juice your grapefruit through a quality juicer, leave the peels on as you juice them, as many of grapefruit's cellulite fighting properties are contained in the white pithy part of the peel.

9. To combat and reverse the signs of sun damage and aging to your skin, here is a highly effective, yet simple to make orange scrub that gently exfoliates away the top

deadened, damaged layers of skin, and stimulates the growth of healthy new skin cells. To make, simply squeeze the juice from 1 large, ripe orange into a small bowl, and slowly add just enough sugar until mixture forms a grainy paste consistency. After freshly washing skin, gently massage the orange scrub onto your facial and neck areas, using small circular motions. Massage for 3-5 minutes, then rinse off with cool water, allow skin to air dry and apply a mineral oil-free moisturizer. The citric acid in the orange is responsible for the exfoliation and stimulation of healthy new skin cells, and gives the added benefit of tightening, toning and brightening your skin. It also helps in cases of mild acne, but for those suffering from acne, always use a very gently massage motion when using a scrub, and do not use more than once a week. For sun damaged and aging skin, you can safely use this scrub 2-3 times a week. If you're just looking to tone and tighten your pores and skin, apply your fresh-squeezed orange juice using a cotton ball directly to your face, and allow to air dry for 5-10 minutes before rinsing with cool water. If you have any skin discolorations, use equal parts fresh lemon juice and fresh orange juice.

10. Fresh oranges are a highly regarded digestive aid, and are one reason why fresh orange wedges are often served along with Chinese dishes. Oranges open up the bowels

and stimulate the flow of digestive juices necessary for proper food assimilation, hastening the passage of food through one's digestive tract for speedy elimination. Eating a few fresh orange wedges is especially helpful after eating a heavy meal, helping to breakdown dietary fats and preventing them from being stored in our arteries and fat tissues.

Cucumbers:

Cucumbers are a favorite salad ingredient for many, and are absolutely bursting with health benefits. So popular are cucumbers, that they are the 4th most cultivated vegetable in the world. Cucumbers belong to the same botanical family as melons, and are commonly divided into two categories: 'slicing cucumbers' (larger and have thicker skin) and 'pickling cucumbers' (smaller and have thinner skin). For a garden variation of Pico de Gallo, swap some cucumbers in place of the jalapeno peppers. Dice up equal parts tomato, red onion and cucumbers, stir in some fresh chopped cilantro, a squeeze of fresh lime juice, and a pinch of garlic powder and sea salt for a fresh garden style Pico de Gallo. When purchasing cucumbers, keep them in the crisper drawer in your fridge to stay crisp, and use within a week.

1. For those who are into all things natural like myself, and like to avoid all chemicals and unnatural ingredients as much as possible, you'll be happy to learn that cucumbers are an effective (and safe) insect repellent for your outdoor gardens and yard areas. If you're looking to repel garden bugs, wasps, mites, moths, flies and other insects, start hanging on to your cucumbers peelings. And, if you have yard areas that seem to be overrun with ants, they are especially turned off by cucumber peels. What I typically do after peeling my cucumbers for a dish, is rough chop the peels then run them for a quick minute in the blender to make grated cucumber peels. This makes it easy to hand spread in my garden, or around the bushes in my front yard where ants love to try and take up residence. I've found that grated cucumber peels work better at repelling those nasty fire ants found here in the southwest desert of Arizona, vs. some of the other natural remedies such as cinnamon. And, if you happen to get stung by a wasp or bee and you have a cucumber on hand, quickly cut up a couple thin slices and place directly over the sting area. You should feel a 'pulling' sensation, as the cucumber works to draw out the sting poison. (please still go to the emergency room, if you feel you are having an allergic reaction – do not wait)

2. Most people already know, that placing some cold fresh cucumber slices over one's

eyes will help reduce puffiness, dark circles and fine lines, as well as refresh tired eyes. But, did you know these same benefits can be had for tired, puffy feet as well? It's true. If you work on your feet all day, and after a long day at work, come home with sweaty, swollen, stinky and oh-so tired feet, you'll want to start regularly keeping cucumbers in the fridge, and use them to make a foot cucumber mash. To make this mash, simply peel 2 large cucumbers, rough chop them, and toss them into a blender. Pulse or puree the cucumbers until smooth, then toss them into a foot bath with cool temperature water. First give your feet a quick wash then plunge them into this soothing cucumber mash foot bath. Relax for 15-30 minutes, then rinse your feet with water before putting on some socks or slippers. You'll notice a difference in your feet after just one use. I used this remedy often when I was working 12 and 24 hours shifts at the hospital, and believe me, it works!

3. Here is a much coveted anti-aging facial mask recipe that I tweaked from a holistic salon for personal use. It's easy to make, and if you apply it 1-2 times a week, you'll be amazed at how it draws out impurities from your pores, tones and tightens skin, hydrates and fills out fine lines and wrinkles, and really gives your skin a bright, radiant glow. To make this mask, peel and chop 2 large cucumbers, and while pureeing, slowly

drizzle in just enough heavy cream till mixture forms a smooth, thick texture, similar to 'Cream-of-Wheat'. Still blending, add in 1 tablespoon olive oil, 1 tablespoon raw honey and a pinch of Bentonite or French face clay. Pour mixture into a container and chill in the fridge for 1 hour. After washing face, first rub half of a sliced lemon across all the areas of your face, neck and décolletage area, or wherever you intend on applying the mask. After the lemon residue air dries, liberally apply the cucumber mask to all your desired skin areas, lay back in a reclining position and allow to sit for 1 full hour before rinsing off with cool water. Do this before bed only, as you don't want to apply any makeup or lotions for at least 8 hours.

4. Cucumbers are high in diuretic and anti-inflammatory properties, making them a great natural remedy to soothe cellular inflammation anywhere in the body. These benefits help reduce acidity and the build-up of crystalline deposits within the body, bringing relief from pain, swelling and stiffness to those suffering from arthritis, gout and rheumatism. Cucumbers will also help flush fluid retention from the body, and is therefore highly beneficial to those suffering from heart and kidney conditions. When you retain fluid, it's not just water. It is water filled with toxic wastes that need to be expelled from the body, but due to

imbalances within the body, is instead being retained. If you suffer from fluid retention, especially if you also have a heart or kidney condition, be sure you're getting lots of fresh cucumbers in your diet.

5. If you are looking for ways to natural lower your elevated blood pressure, cucumbers can help you do just that. Just 1 cup of cucumbers contains 16 micrograms of magnesium and 181 mg of potassium, necessary minerals that your body needs to keep your blood pressure within a healthy range. And, cucumbers contain the hard-to-find vitamin K, a vitamin necessary for maintaining bone density and good bone health, which can reduce your risk of osteoporosis, arthritis and other bone degenerative conditions.

Figs:

While you can find dried figs at your local market any time of the year, there's something about the sweetness of a fresh fig that you can't get when eating a dried fig. I'm lucky enough to have a fig tree in my backyard, and I get to enjoy ample amounts of fresh figs all summer long. Fresh California figs are available during the summer months, and fresh European figs are typically available during the autumn months. And, when it comes to that sweetness factor, figs have the highest sugar content of common fruits, so for those concerned with high blood sugar or candida, it's best just to use figs for topical purposes only, to avoid aggravating any existing conditions. Additionally, figs contain a natural occurring compound called 'oxalate'. When oxalates become concentrated in body fluids, they can crystallize and cause health problems for those with existing or untreated kidney or gallbladder conditions. So, for those individuals, it's best to avoid figs all together.

1. As long as you don't have any blood sugar or candida issues, figs should be a top priority food for those looking to prevent or remedy cancer. While absolutely no claims are being made, figs have been used throughout the world to combat cancer. Figs possess 2 important compounds that are responsible for this. The first is polyphenols, which are natural chemicals found in plants, and are said to help reduce the risk of cancer. And, figs happen to be a very rich source of these important polyphenols. Secondly, figs contain cancer-fighting 'benzaldehyde', a compound researchers have proven to have the ability to shrink abnormal growths.

2. For those suffering from the painful symptoms of arthritis, gout or rheumatism, as well as those who are looking to bring

their body into a healthy, slightly alkaline range, you'll definitely want to regularly add some figs to your diet. Figs are highly alkaline and not only help to bring the body back into a healthy pH range, they also help reduce acidic waste build-up in the body, especially the acidic crystalline waste accumulation found in the joints of those suffering from arthritis and other similar conditions, helping to bring relief from pain, swelling and stiffness. Suggested dosage is 2 fresh or dried figs daily.

3. Figs make an excellent poultice to draw out infection and other toxins from skin conditions such as boils, carbuncles, warts, blisters, ulcerations, abnormal skin growths and insect bites. To make a poultice using fresh figs, first heat 1 or more gently in the oven or a saucepan (never use the microwave, as this irradiates food & beverage and removes all nutrients and other beneficial properties). Remove from heat, and slice each fig in half. Lay the fig, cut-side down against the affected skin areas, and secure in place with medical tape, gauze, or a handkerchief. Replace with a fresh fig poultice every 8 hours, and use until condition clears. To make a poultice using dried figs, first soften 1 or more figs in some hot water. Remove from water and slice in half. Apply figs cut-side down against affected skin areas and secure. Results may take longer to notice when

using dried figs instead of fresh figs. I used this remedy once to rid a small wart on my granddaughter's foot. It worked just as well as a banana peel, and was a little easier to keep in place on her small foot.

4. Figs also are great for natural teeth and gum care. You can actually effectively and gently, clean your teeth using fresh cut figs, and that's exactly what many people do in Africa, Central America and other parts of the world, to keep their teeth clean. After cutting a fig in half, rub the cut-side against your teeth in a back-and-forth motion for several minutes, and then rinse with a mouthful of water. Figs anti-inflammatory properties also make it a great remedy for teeth and gum abscesses, helping to bring you relief until you can get to a dentist. Simply rub a cut fig across the affected tooth or gum area, until a layer of fig residue remains. Do not rinse mouth. Instead, allow residue to remain as long as possible and avoiding eating or drinking anything for 1 hour.

5. Both fresh and dried figs are rich in dietary fiber, and act as a safe and gentle laxative with no unwanted side effects. And, for people who just have trouble digesting beans, and tend to get excess gas when consuming them, figs might be a better dietary choice for making sure you are consuming enough dietary fiber in your diet.

Dietary fiber is always better than fiber supplements, because it is naturally occurring and your body knows what to do with dietary fiber. Fiber supplements aren't natural to the human body, and are the reason why many people often get aggravated digestive symptoms instead of alleviated symptoms when using them, so it's always best to get your fiber from dietary sources vs. supplements. Aim to eat 1 fresh or dried fig a day for digestive health.

Garlic:

While I don't know the success rate of how well garlic does to repel vampires, werewolves and other demons, I do know that garlic IS very successful at repelling undesirable foreign invaders within the body. Part of the onion family, garlic has been used for centuries in traditional Chinese medicine, herbal medicine, folk medicine and on just about every continent across the globe. Garlic's therapeutic powers are vast, and thankfully fresh garlic is no more than a quick trip to your local market. When purchasing fresh garlic, you want to select cloves that are firm with lots of dry 'papery' covering and have no sprouts coming from them. The best way to store fresh garlic is in a cool, dry, dark place with ventilation. You do not want to store fresh garlic in the fridge, because it is likely to get soft and moldy. You also do NOT want to store fresh garlic in oil, as this can lead to botulism. The very best way to store fresh garlic is to invest in a garlic storing container made of ceramic, which will have ventilation holes around the top. They are inexpensive and a 'must-have' for your kitchen needs. What about pre-minced garlic you find in the market in the produce section? I highly recommend avoiding them, and stick to fresh garlic for both your cooking and natural remedy needs.

1. Probably the very best characteristic of fresh garlic, is that it is Mother Nature's broad-spectrum natural antibiotic. Garlic is rich with antiviral, antibacterial, antifungal and anti-parasitic properties, making it a powerful dietary staple for the prevention, healing and recovery of colds, flu, intestinal parasites and other unwanted 'bugs'. As recently as just a few generations ago, our ancestors were very aware of the healing properties of fresh garlic, and in addition to all the above mentioned benefits, fresh garlic was routinely hung in areas where patients were conflicted with conditions such as the plague, and tuberculosis, to cleanse the area of airborne pathogens, helping to contain and prevent the spread of contaminated air particles. To use during cold and flu season, or to help heal through a digestive complaint such as parasites or food

poisoning, make a tea by steeping 1 fresh garlic clove (sliced – to release the garlic oils) in a cup of freshly boiled water for 5 minutes. Strain out the garlic, and stir in a squeeze of fresh lemon juice and 1 teaspoon of raw honey. Drink a cup every couple hours during acute healing phases, every 4-6 hours during tolerable healing phases, and then once day or every other day for prevention during cold and flu season. (Yes, you can add a shot of brandy into the tea if desired.) You can also include lots of fresh garlic into your dishes as well, but refrain from eating raw garlic, as this will be too caustic on your digestive system, and can cause ulcerations if done too often.

2. If you are a gardener, here's a chemical-free insecticide recipe developed by a horticulture group in California, which produced astonishing results. To make, finely mince a handful of fresh garlic cloves and soak them in mineral oil for a full 24 hours. Spoon out 2 tablespoons of this garlic-infused mineral oil, and add it to 1 pint (16 ounces) of water. Then add in 2-1/4 tablespoon of dishwashing liquid (their recipe specifically uses Palmolive brand), and gently shake until all ingredients are thoroughly combined. This now becomes your insecticide concentrate. To now make it into a spray that you can use to spray your garden plants with, combine 2 tablespoon of this concentrate with 1 pint of water (16

ounces) in a spray bottle. Be sure to label and cover with a clear, moisture-proof tape. This recipe reportedly kills cabbage moths, cabbage loopers, earwigs, potato bugs, grasshoppers, mosquitoes (including larvae), whiteflies and some aphids on contact. Houseflies, June bugs and squash bugs typically die within minutes after being sprayed, and cockroaches, slugs and hornworms die more slowly.

3. Garlic is also incredibly beneficial for heart health, and helping to keep blood pressure within a more normal range. One of the reasons is due to garlic's natural sulfur compounds called 'polysulfides'. Our red blood cells uptake these polysulfides, and use them to produce hydrogen sulfide (H2S), which in turn helps our blood vessels to expand and keep our blood pressure in check. Interestingly, yet not surprising, some processed garlic extracts cannot be used by our red blood cells in this way, and do not seem to provide the same level of cardiac protection that fresh garlic in food form can.

4. It might surprise you to learn, that consuming fresh garlic regularly can have a positive effect on your weight. To help explain, researchers classify obesity as a chronic state of cellular inflammation. Furthermore, researchers clarify that some of our fibroblastic cells only evolve into full-fledged fat cells under certain metabolic

conditions involving inflammatory system activity. Consuming fresh garlic with natural sulfur compounds (1,2-DT; 1,2-vinyldithiin) that have high anti-inflammatory properties, helps fend off this inflammatory cell response, that might otherwise convert certain body cells into full-fledged fat cells. In simpler terms, garlic's unique sulfur compounds help to prevent the conversion and formation of fat cells within the body.

5. To help clear up chest and lung congestion overnight, here is a simple garlic-oil recipe to use for just such an occasion. Slice up several fresh garlic cloves and soak them in 2 ounces of olive, coconut or almond oil. Allow to stand for 1 hour or more. Using a basting brush or plastic gloves on your hands, spread a liberal amount of this garlic-infused oil across the soles of both feet, then put on some old, heavy socks. Keep them on while you sleep. In the morning, wash off with warm, soapy water. You should notice a slight garlic odor to your breath. Garlic oil applied this way, enters your system and heads straight for your lungs, and goes to work quickly to help break up and dispel lodged mucus from your lungs and chest, allow you to cough, sneeze and expel this pathogen-infused fluid from your body with ease. My grandmother showed me this trick when I was a new mother, and I used it often on my kids whenever they started to get a little cold. I can tell you, it worked

amazingly fast, and always prevented those sniffles from manifesting into a full blown cold.

6. Garlic kills yeast like crazy, and bakers know that you can't add garlic to bread or pastry dough until after it has risen, because it will kill the yeast and prevent the dough from rising. If you're a woman and suffer from yeast infections, if you catch it in its early stages, garlic can knock it down before the yeast takes hold and becomes widespread in your body. In fact, this garlic remedy can knock out a new yeast infection within 1-2 days, and often just overnight. Before bed, peel the papery layers from 1 clove of fresh garlic. Do not slice or mash. Insert the garlic clove whole into the vagina, and leave in overnight while you're sleeping. In the morning, discard the garlic clove in the toilet when you urinate, then take a shower or bath. The garlic often causes a watery discharge during this remedy, so it's advisable to put down a large old towel over your bedding while sleeping. If you notice a slight garlic taste in your mouth in the morning, you know the garlic did its job. Never, ever douche when you have a yeast infection, as yeast loves water, and this only causes the yeast to multiply, thereby making the problem worse. You can still use this remedy for more severe cases of yeast infection, but it might take several days to notice relief. By the way, this natural

yeast remedy has been used by holistic veterinarians in livestock for decades, if not hundreds of years.

7. Here's another natural weight loss remedy using fresh garlic. Garlic's properties help pull excess sugar out of the blood. Adding some fresh garlic to a morning weight loss elixir consisting of warm water, fresh lime juice and a pinch of black pepper can help boost your weight loss efforts by 50%. Just combine ½ of a clove of fresh garlic (minced) with the juice of 1 large lime, 8 ounces of filtered water and a pinch of black pepper in a blender, and blend for 30-60 seconds on high. Drink each morning within 30 minutes of rising on an empty stomach, and wait an additional 30 minutes before eating or drinking anything else.

8. To make an everyday garlic tonic, that you can take each morning to help maintain good health and fend off infection, heart ailments, skin problems, weight gain, female complaints, urinary disorders, diseases of the brain such as Alzheimer's and even cancer, here's a recipe that you can make on a weekly basis, will last you 5-7 days, and should be kept in the fridge during that time. In a blender, combine 8 cloves of fresh garlic (sliced or minced for easy blending), 1 cup raw honey (do NOT use processed honey ever), and 1 cup pure apple cider vinegar with the 'mother'. (the 'mother'

means it is unfiltered and will still have the floating live enzymes in the container). Puree mixture for 1-2 minutes, then transfer into a sealable glass jar, and keep in the fridge. Suggested dosage is 2 teaspoons of this garlic tonic in a glass of water or juice each morning on an empty stomach, waiting 30 minutes before consuming any food or beverage.

9. The same garlic-oil recipe that was described above to break up chest and lung congestion can also be used to bring quick relief from earaches and ear infection. Take 1-2 fresh cloves of garlic (sliced or minced), and put into 2 ounces of olive, coconut or almond oil, and allow to stand for 1 hour or more, so the garlic's healing anti-inflammatory, antifungal, antiviral and antibacterial properties infuse into the oil. When suffering from an earache, swimmers ear, or a possible ear infection, drizzle a few drops of the garlic-infused oil into the affected ear, and gently massage into the ear while either resting your head on the unaffected side, or on your back if both ears are affected. This should bring slight relief within 30 minutes, and much-improved (if not complete) relief within a couple hours or so. As always, this does not negate a possible need to see your doctor, but it is a very tried-and true remedy that has brought relief from earaches and infections for centuries.

10. If you want to heal a cold sore on the inside of your mouth or on your lips fast, AND you can tolerate a little bit of discomfort, a fresh garlic clove can bring speedy healing to those cold sores. First gargle with some warm water that has a pinch of real sea salt in it (NEVER use table salt for anything), to cleanse the mouth of residual debris. Slice a fresh garlic clove in half, and hold cut-side down onto the cold sore for 5 minutes. (This is when you'll typically feel some stinging, but try to bear with it.) Discard the halved garlic clove and refrain from eating or drinking anything for the next hour. Garlic's antiviral, antibacterial and antiseptic properties are now going to work, to bring fast relief and healing to that cold sore, significantly reducing its duration and discomfort. If you catch a cold sore early enough, when you can't see it yet, but feel some tingling in the area, try this garlic remedy, to prevent the cold sore from breaking out in the first place.

Ginger:

Next to garlic and lemon, fresh ginger root is a Veggie Goddess favorite, and is abundant in both flavor and uses. Ginger is a staple ingredient to Asian cuisine and can easily be found year-round in your local market. When you purchase fresh ginger root, it's best stored in a paper bag placed in the crisper drawer of your fridge. A chunk of ginger root will stay fresh this way for up to 2 weeks. And, for easy peeling, just scrape the thin outer skin off with the edge of a spoon. A very effective, yet little known characteristic of fresh ginger, is its ability to interfere with cholesterol biosynthesis, which means it natural helps to lower serum cholesterol, without the dangerous side effects of cholesterol lowering drugs.

1. There is absolutely nothing like fresh ginger to calm a myriad of digestive complaints. From preventing sea sickness, to squashing nausea, vomiting, heartburn, excess gas and bloating, ginger is your 'go-to' for quick digestive relief. Ginger has a very unique component called 'gingerol', which helps block serotonin receptors in the stomach that cause nausea and can lead to vomiting. Fresh ginger has even proved to be more effective than the popular over-the-counter medicine Dramamine in reducing the incidence of nausea and vomiting due to sea sickness. Fresh ginger root tea is often given to cancer patients in holistic cancer centers, for the prevention of chemotherapy-induced nausea. To make ginger tea, grate 1 teaspoon of fresh ginger root into a large cup, and pour 8 ounces of boiling over it. Allow the ginger to steep for 5 minutes, and

then strain out the grated ginger pieces. You can enjoy the tea 'as-is', or add a pinch of fresh squeezed lemon, raw honey or stevia to adjust the flavor as needed. While ginger tea is typically safe even for pregnant women to use, please consult with your doctor before using.

2. Ginger is also quite effective in supporting cardiac health. Ginger contains 2 important compounds called 'Terpenes' and 'Oleoresin', and both of these compounds possess antiseptic, anti-inflammatory, blood vessel dilating and circulation promoting properties. For this reason, ginger has proven to be as effective in inhibiting the blood thickening enzyme as aspirin is, but without the side effects associated with long-term use of aspiring, including stomach bleeding. Consuming fresh ginger root regularly helps to keep blood vessels dilated, thin the blood, and help keep blood pressure within a lower, healthier range. If you currently take heart medications, including blood thinners and cholesterol lowering drugs, do not stop taking them without first consulting with your doctor about consuming ginger.

3. In today's modern world, fibromyalgia is a condition that is affecting people at an almost epidemic rate, and those who suffer with this condition struggle with pain on a daily basis. An alternative to swallowing a

steady stream of over-the-counter or prescription pain medication, and then dealing with the unwanted side effects such as rebound pain, stomach bleeding, liver dysfunction and addiction, is to take dried ginger as a safer alternative for pain relief. Fibromyalgia patients have elevated amounts of a pain mediator known as 'Substance P'. Dried ginger, unlike its fresh counterpart, contains a compound known as 'shogaol', which has been proven to effectively inhibit this 'Substance P', in those suffering from fibromyalgia-related pain. Suggested dosage is 1000 mg of dried ginger daily for mild pain symptoms and 3,000-4,000 mg daily for quicker and even more effective relief.

4. Whenever you have a cold, flu or other type of 'bug', here is a tried-and-true effective 'Hot Toddy' recipe that you'll love after just one try. Grate 1 teaspoon of fresh ginger root into a large mug. Pour 8-10 ounces of boiling water into the mug, cover the mug with a small plate, and let steep for 5-7 minutes. Stir in 1 teaspoon raw honey (never use processed honey), fresh squeezed juice from ½ half of a lemon, a pinch of cayenne pepper, and 1 shot (or 2!) of brandy. Ginger's natural antibiotic, antibacterial, antiviral and antiseptic properties will not only help kill the pathogens that have caused the cold or flu, but it will also bring you relief from pain, congestion and digestive

upset. The fresh lemon, raw honey and cayenne also contribute their potent antiviral, antibacterial properties, while the brandy offers both antiseptic and anesthetic properties to the toddy. Together, these 'Hot Toddy' ingredients can bring you much needed, quick relief from your symptoms, while also shortening the duration of your illness.

5. A rather unknown remedy using fresh ginger is in the use of various skin healing needs. Gently anointing minor skin burns and skin rashes, has proven to greatly hasten their healing, while at the same time reducing the incidence and severity of scarring. Fresh ginger can also be used for older scars with positive results. For either case, simply slice off a piece of fresh ginger and rub gently across the affected area until you notice a light residue on the skin area. Do not wash off, and instead allow the residue to air dry on the skin. Rinse with cool water after 4 hours, and keep area exposed to air as often as possible. Results can start to be seen within days, and in cases of older scars, you should notice an improvement within 6-12 weeks with once a day use.

Grapes:

Grapes have a unique flavor combination of sweet and tart, are made up of 65%-85% water and 10%-33% sugar (depending on the variety). The Fox grape variety is what kept the Lewis and Clark Expedition from near starvation. While grapes are delicious and healthy, if you have an unfilled cavity in any of your teeth, eating grapes, or drinking grape juice, can intensify tooth destruction, so be sure to rinse your mouth with water after eating grapes. And, if you've ever gotten an upset stomach after eating grapes, it may just have been due to a bad food combination. To avoid upset stomach, do NOT eat grapes with milk products, mineral water, beer, fish, cucumbers, any type of melon, or fatty meals. When purchasing grapes, choose 'bunches' with firm stems, and fruit that is firm and without bruising, tears or wrinkles. Do not ever wash grapes before storing, as this can actually make the mushy and promote bacterial growth on the outer skins. Keep them stored in a tightly sealed Ziploc bag or plastic storage container, and they will keep fresh for a week.

1. Oregon grapes are especially beneficially in the prevention and treatment of colds, flu, food poisoning and other 'bugs'. The berberine alkaloid, a constituent of Oregon grapes, inhibits the ability of bacteria to

attach to human cells, which helps prevent and treat infections. In research studies, Oregon grapes have been shown to kill or suppress even the nastiest of pathogens, including E.coli, Candida, Giardia Lamblia, Streptococcus, Staphylococcus, Trichomonas Vaginalis, Vibrio Cholerae and numerous others. If you feel you are coming down with a 'bug', start eating 1 cup of Oregon grapes daily, to prevent the 'bug' from taking hold. If you've already caught the 'bug', start eating 2 cups of Oregon grapes daily, along with lots of alkalizing vegetables and plenty of fresh water to shorten the duration of your illness, relieve symptoms and hasten recovery.

2. To support those who are recovering alcoholics and are going through recovery, drinking pure Oregon grape juice will help support the return of your health. The same berberine alkaloids found in Oregon grapes that prevent and treat infections, also acts as a bitter tonic, stimulating the flow of bile and intestinal secretions, improving both digestive health and liver function in recovering alcohols. These berberine alkaloids have even been shown to be of benefit to those who already have cirrhosis of the liver. In addition, these same alkaloids prove to also be beneficial in treating jaundice and hepatitis.

3. For matters of anti-aging skin care, holistic

spas and salons have long used fresh grapes in their spa therapies, especially for the treatment of fine lines, wrinkles, sagging crepey skin, and age spots. Fresh grapes are loaded with alpha-hydroxy acids, which work to natural exfoliate skin, and stimulate the rejuvenation of healthy new skin cells. They are also rich in important minerals and antioxidants, which help support collagen production, and protect against the damaging effects of too much sun and other free radical skin damage. One easy grape remedy to help reduce crows-feet and fine line around the mouth, is to cut a few rip grapes in half, and rub the cut-side across any areas where you have fine lines and wrinkles, until you have a nice layer of grape juice residue on the skin. Let the grape residue sit for 30 minutes, then rinse with cool water and apply a mineral oil-free moisturizer. For a more intensified anti-again grape mask remedy, try the following recipe. In a blender, combine 1 cup of fresh grapes, 2 teaspoons olive oil, ¼ cup heavy cream (you may also substitute with plain yogurt), and ½ teaspoon of baking soda. Blend until mixture is smooth, and apply in an even layer to freshly washed skin on your face and neck. Leave on for 30 minutes, and then rinse mixture off with cool water.

4. And, grapes bestow more than just anti-aging skin care benefits our way, they also have other anti-aging benefits, such as

preventing age-related diseases and illnesses such as heart conditions, stroke, Alzheimer's disease and more. Eating fresh grapes promotes healthy digestion, stamina, protection against illness and longevity. The polyphenols, minerals, antioxidants and other phytonutrients found in grapes (mostly in the skin, followed by the seeds, then the flesh), have been proven to increase expression of 3 different gene markers specifically related to longevity. These 3 gene markers are SirT1s, FoxOs, and PBEFs. The enormous amount of antioxidants and anti-inflammatories found in fresh grapes also makes for great nutritional protection against cancer, because chronic oxidative stress and chronic inflammation are key factors in the development of cancer. For the prevention of age-related illnesses and diseases and general anti-aging benefits, aim to eat ½ cup of fresh grapes, or 6 ounces of pure (no added sugar or additional ingredients) grape juice daily.

5. There are many protocol options for detoxification of the body, and eating grapes is one such options. Our bodies are constantly being assaulted with environmental pollutants, chemicals from the foods we eat, and absorbed through our skin via commercial toiletries. We constantly need to cleanse our body to purge out this toxic waste buildup, which left unchecked, leads to unresolved weight gain,

skin disorders, depression and other health concerns. Here is a protocol you can follow for NO LONGER than 6 days, and it's best advised to start with a single day or 2 or 3 day protocol, preferably over a weekend, before you try to do a full 6 days. To ease into the protocol, avoid heavy meals for 3 days prior to starting. You also want to avoid caffeine and alcohol. For each day you are on the detox protocol, you will eat a 'bunch' of green or purple grapes every 2-3 hours, for a total of 6 grape servings a day. You also need to drink a minimum of 8 full glasses of pure water, and relax as much as you can, so as not to divert your body's energies which are focusing on cleansing, repairing and rejuvenating your body's tissues. You can expect to need to use the bathroom frequently, as your body is purging these toxins from your digestive system. In addition to losing some excess pounds, you should notice an improvement in sleep, mental clarity, mood and stamina. When you finish the duration of your grape detox, do not re-pollute your body by filling it with junk food. Eat a light, healthy meal consisting of lots of fresh vegetables.

Honey:

For all these honey recipes, including the mentioning of honey as an addition to any other remedy in this book, as well as any recipe within any of my vegetarian and vegan cookbooks, it will ALWAYS only refer to RAW honey. This is crucial folks. Raw honey means that it is unfiltered, unprocessed, unpasteurized and unheated. Raw honey is brimming with vitamins, minerals, antioxidants, live enzymes and so much more. It is very alkalizing to the body, and will always have a natural grainy, crystallized look to it. Processed honey on the other hand, is not fit for human consumption, as the pasteurization and processing of the honey react with the honey in such a way, that when the honey is consumed it becomes more like glue in our body, and is devoid of its natural nutrients and enzymes. Studies have even uncovered that most processed honey found in commercial markets actually consists of a corn syrup mixture. No truth in advertising here folks, and this is where being informed can help you make better decisions when it comes to your health and well-being. WARNING: Never give honey to a child under 2 years of age.

1. When raw honey is combined with organic cinnamon, it creates a very healing mixture that can be used topically as a salve.

Cinnamon's essential oils, and honey's enzyme that produces hydrogen peroxide, combine to produce anti-microbial properties that help stop the growth of bacteria as well as fungi. Combine ½ a teaspoon of pure organic cinnamon with ¼ cup of raw honey, and keep it in a small container to use as a healing skin salve. Use this honey cinnamon salve for skin wounds, minor burns, acne, skin rashes and more. Do NOT use honey for diaper rash problems, or skin problems in the genital areas, as this is a moist, warm area of the body that will act like a petri dish in the lab, causing the natural sugar molecules in the honey to turn into a yeast outbreak. As long as you keep the container with the honey salve tightly sealed, it will literally last forever.

2. If you have gum disease, you know that staying away from processed sugars is a must for teeth and gum health. However, the exception to that rule is raw honey, and more specifically, Manuka raw honey. As already mentioned, honey has a unique enzyme that produces hydrogen peroxide, which is believed to be the key reason for the antimicrobial properties of honey. For this reason, raw honey actually helps prevent dental plaque bacteria growth, as well as reduces the amount of acid produced, which stops the bacteria from producing dextran, a component of dental plaque that adheres stubbornly to the surface

of teeth. All raw honey provides this benefit, but Manuka raw honey was proven to possess double the amount of this unique enzyme, and in lab studies Manuka honey was found to be as effective as the standard antiseptic phenol. To use raw honey for the healing and prevention of gum disease, just rub a dab across your top and bottom gums after brushing your teeth, and refrain from eating or drinking anything for 30 minutes.

3. Honey can also be used as a natural remedy in the thickening of thin hair, preventing hair loss, rejuvenating the scalp and encouraging hair growth. To make this honey hair tonic, stir together 1 heaping tablespoon of raw honey with ¼ cup fresh onion juice. Massage thoroughly into your scalp, cover with a shower cap, and leave on overnight. Shampoo your hair in the morning, and always do a final rinse of your hair with cold water, to seal the outer hair cuticles. You can also substitute pure aloe vera juice or gel in place of the raw onion juice, but results are said to be better using the onion juice.

4. When it comes to easing the discomfort of a sore, scratchy throat, or calming a hacking cough, raw honey is packed with antibacterial, antiviral, antiseptic and antimicrobial properties that bring rapid relief from symptoms and speed healing. Rather than use a chemical-laden commercial cough syrup, try this homemade

honey cough syrup instead. In a small bowl, stir together 1 tablespoon raw honey, ¼ teaspoon cayenne pepper, ¼ teaspoon powdered ginger, 1 tablespoon apple cider vinegar (do not consume white vinegar) and 2 tablespoons water. Once well blended, consume your homemade throat and cough syrup. Repeat every 4 hours during acute phases, and less frequently for milder cases.

5. Want a sure-fire remedy to combat those stubborn fine lines and wrinkles? Who doesn't? Raw honey is not only bursting with nutrients that rejuvenate skin cells, it is also a natural humectant, meaning it causes skin tissue to hold in moisture. Using raw honey on your face, neck and décolletage area will help slough off dead skin cells, and plump up skin with much-needed moisture, helping to smooth away those fine lines and wrinkles. To use, simply spread a thin layer of raw honey onto desired areas after washing skin. Lay back and allow honey to set on skin for 30 minutes, and then rinse off with cold water. Allow your face to air dry. For maximum wrinkle-fighting benefits, do at least 3 times a week. This is so easy to fit into your skin care routine, and you'll be amazed at how radiant your skin will start to look.

6. In today's chaotic times, it seems that almost everyone is plagued with sleep disturbance either on a regular basis, or intermittently.

Sleep is absolutely vital to one's health and well-being, and there is no badge of honor for how long you can go without sleep. During sleep, our bodies are hard at work repairing, rejuvenating and balancing all of our cells, and every time we fail to get an adequate amount of sleep, instead of our bodies repairing and rejuvenating our bodies, a cascade of stress signals flood the body with stress hormones that actually prevent our bodies from repairing themselves. Sleep disturbances cause stubborn weight gain that you can't get rid of, mood swings, depression, chronic fatigue and so much more. Left unchecked, it goes on to potentially manifest into more serious health conditions. Everyone's grandma knew the best remedy to help you fall asleep....a spoonful of honey. Typically our grandmas would stir it into a glass of warm milk, but that was back in the days when raw milk was delivered to your doorstep. And, unlike pasteurized milk, occasionally drinking raw milk was actually good for you. So, in place of body-harming pasteurized milk, if you're having trouble falling asleep or staying asleep, simply drink a small glass of warm water with 1-2 teaspoons of raw honey stirred into it. Sweet dreams.

7. If you suffer from bad breath due to eating pungent foods, smoking, drinking coffee or alcohol, in addition to brushing your teeth

after every meal try rinsing your mouth out with this highly effective breath-freshening honey concoction. Stir in 1 teaspoon of raw honey and 1/8 teaspoon organic cinnamon powder into a glass of warm water, and after brushing your teeth, gargle and swish this mixture around in your mouth for a full 1-2 minutes. The strong antibacterial and antimicrobial properties in this honey mixture effectively kill halitosis (bad breath)-causing germs, helping to keep your breath clean and fresh. Gargling with this mixture will also help to heal and prevent bleeding gums, and prevent tooth decay.

8. Here's a great honey remedy that will help fade and diminish scars that are a result of acne, chicken pox, surgical cuts and all those nicks and dings we tend to give ourselves over the course of our lifetime. Stir together ½ teaspoon of ground nutmeg with 1 teaspoon of raw honey. After washing face, apply a thin layer to scar-affected areas, and let set on skin for 30-60 minutes before rinsing off with cool water. Immediately after rinsing, apply some pure aloe vera gel to your face, and avoid wearing makeup for the next several hours. For this reason, it's best to use this honey remedy before bed. The more often you do this, the quicker the scars will fade.

9. These days, there are far too many people reaching for unhealthy 'energy drinks' that

are being heavily promoted. They are loaded with stuff you don't want to be consuming, are potentially dangerous to your health, and expensive on the pocketbook. To make your own healthy energy drink, that's brimming with electrolytes, natural, easy-to-digest sugars and lots of fresh flavor, try the following recipe. (I recommend making this in larger batches, and keeping it in a pitcher in the fridge so you'll always have some on hand.) Grate a 2 inch piece of fresh ginger root, and place in 2 quarts of filtered water. Place in fridge for 3 hours or so, to allow the natural oils in the ginger to infuse the water. Strain out the ginger, and stir in 3-4 tablespoons of raw honey, the freshly-squeezed juice of 2 limes and an optional pinch of cayenne pepper. Shake or stir to blend, and your healthy, honey energy drink is ready to drink.

10. Arthritis, osteoarthritis and rheumatoid arthritis are very common complaints today, and for those suffering from any of these conditions, you know all too well the pain and stiffness you have to deal with is no walk in the park. Raw honey's strong anti-inflammatory properties are very beneficial in helping to reduce inflammation within and around joints, thereby relieving pain in these areas and improving your range of motion and mobility. To consume honey for this purpose, first brew a large cup of green tea. Stir in 2 teaspoons of raw honey and ½

teaspoon organic cinnamon powder. Drink this 2-3 times a day for relief of your symptoms. A note about purchasing green tea. It's best purchased in powdered form from a reputable vendor. Green tea bags that are typically purchased in stores have already oxidized, which is indicated by the brown leaf color. This discoloration indicates that the healing properties in the green tea have deteriorated. Green tea should always appear bright green in color.

Kiwis:

A single kiwi packs more vitamin C than an orange, and more potassium than a large banana. Kiwis have a unique sweet flavor profile to them, and are full of health benefits. Even those tiny black seeds in the center of the fruit, contain Alfa-Linoleic Acid, an important Omega-3 essential fatty acid. Be cautious when consuming the first couple times, especially small children, since there is a percentage of the population that is allergic to kiwis. Kiwis contain a protein-dissolving enzyme called 'actinidin', which is responsible for these allergic reactions. Symptoms include itching and swelling of the lips, tongue and palate, and the most severe symptoms include wheezing, shortness of breath and swelling of the airways. If you ever feel like you're having an allergic reaction to kiwis (or any other food), do not wait it out. Immediately call 911. When purchasing kiwi, they should feel firm, but give slightly with a gentle squeeze. Avoid specimens with bruising, tears, or skin wrinkling. Kiwis will stay fresh at room temperature for a few days, and up to 2 weeks when stored inside a crisper drawer in the fridge.

1. Kiwi contains natural fruit acids that make a gentle, yet highly effective skin exfoliator. Unlike harsh chemical peels, unless you are allergic to kiwis, you can safely use them as an anti-aging skin remedy several times a week, to keep your skin taught, vibrant and wrinkle-free. To make this kiwi skin mask, simply combine 2 peeled, diced kiwi and 5 de-stemmed strawberries in a blender, and puree until smooth. Transfer into a small bowl, and stir in 1-2 teaspoons of rolled oats (uncooked), until mixture is thickened. After washing face and neck area, spread on an even layer of this kiwi skin mask to all of the skin areas you with to cover, including your face, neck and décolletage region. Lay back and let mixture stand for 30 minutes, then rinse off with cool water and apply a mineral oil-free moisturizer. If you don't have sensitive skin, and desire a more intense exfoliating treatment, after washing face, do a gentle sugar scrub to your skin areas before applying the mask. Just put about a quarter-size amount of sugar into

your hands, and drizzle just a few drops of water into the sugar to make a paste-like consistency. Using the pads of your fingers, use small circular motions for 1-2 minutes, to do a pre-exfoliating treatment. Rinse off sugar, allow skin to air dry, and apply the kiwi skin mask. You might feel some slight stinging the first minute or two, and if it's too much, just rinse with cool water. If you decide to do the more intense exfoliating treatment, only do this 1-2 times a week at most.

2. For those suffering from IBS (irritable bowel syndrome), the symptoms are a constant oscillation of diarrhea, constipation, bloating and gas. Symptoms often affect one's lifestyle, and quality of life. The good news is, researchers have discovered that IBS patients who consumed 2 fresh kiwis daily, had a marked reduction in their symptoms after just 30 days. Eating kiwi seemed to help IBS sufferers who suffered primarily from constipation the most, followed by those primarily complaining of excess gas and bloating. Apparently, the fruit fiber contained in kiwis is gentle enough to the digestive system of IBS sufferers to not further aggravate their symptoms, while at the same time, effective enough to reduce their symptoms and discomfort.

3. For those suffering from mild hypertension,

eating 3 fresh kiwis daily has been proven effective at lowering one's blood pressure readings. Credit goes to several factors. First, kiwi has diuretic properties, which helps to naturally flush stored toxic fluid build-up from the body. Secondly, kiwi is rich in potassium, a mineral crucial to the balancing and normalization of blood pressure. And thirdly, one of kiwi's unique antioxidants is 'lutein', a carotenoid that helps prevent the build-up of plaque within the arteries. So, while an apple-a-day still helps to keep the doctor away, consuming 3 kiwis a day will also help keep high blood pressure away as well.

4. Kiwis contain a rich variety of flavonoids and carotenoids. These potent phytonutrients have shown to be beneficial in reducing the occurrence and severity of respiratory-related illnesses, including asthma. Researchers discovered that symptoms such as wheezing, shortness of breath and night coughing were all able to be reduced when as little as 3 fresh kiwi were eaten per week, on a regular basis. The highest benefits came to those who ate 5-7 kiwis per week on a regular basis. For those individuals, there was a 44% reduction in wheezing; a 32% reduction in shortness of breath; a 41% reduction in night coughing; a 25% reduction in chronic cough; and a 28% reduction in runny nose.

5. The Archives of Ophthalmology declare that eating certain fresh fruits, is an effective and healthy way to naturally lowering your risk of age-related macular degeneration. Kiwi just so happens to be one of those fruits beneficial to eye health, because it is loaded with all the right nutrients that our eyes need. In fact, controlled studies have proven that eating 3 kiwis a day helped reduce age-related macular degeneration for an impressive 36% of the study participants, over participants that only consumed 1 serving a day.

Leafy Greens:

I can't emphasize enough, the importance of including lots of fresh leafy greens into your diet. While all fruits and vegetables offer amazing health, weight loss and beauty benefits, dark, leafy greens rank #1 in the all-inclusive nutrient department. Dark leafy greens support your immune system better than drugs, facilitate detoxification and healthy weight loss of our bodies better than dangerous pills or crash diets, and provide so many vital nutrients, that you can forego buying expensive supplements. And, unlike some fruits and vegetables, almost nobody experiences an allergic reaction to eating dark leafy greens. The best way to store leafy greens is to wash them in cold water, pat them mostly dry, and then wrap them in a single layer of paper towels. Next, place them in a plastic grocery bag, and store them in the crisper drawer in your fridge. This should help keep your greens fresh for up to a week. Never purchase more greens than you'll use within the next 5-7 days.

1. Eating steamed collard greens has been proven to be a powerful and natural way to lower one's levels of bad cholesterol (LDL). Once consumed, the collard greens go to work binding to bile acids within the digestive tract, making it easier for them to be expelled from the body. Since bile acids are made from cholesterol stores within the body, the net impact of this bile acid binding is a natural lowering of the body's cholesterol level. When consuming collard greens for cholesterol-lowering effects, researchers found that these benefits were realized when eating collard greens steamed vs. eating them raw.

2. When it comes to preventing, controlling and reducing the dangerous side effects of diabetes and metabolic syndrome (also known as insulin resistance and 'Syndrome X'), Swiss chard is one mean, green blood sugar balancing machine. Swiss chard is packed with phytonutrient goodness, including at least 13 different polyphenol antioxidants, and an untold number of

flavonoids, including its primary flavonoid 'syringic acid'. This flavonoid has been shown to inhibit activity of an enzyme called 'alpha-glucosidase'. When this enzyme gets inhibited, fewer carbohydrates are broken down into simple sugars, helping to keep blood sugar levels steady.

3. Mustard greens are an often overlooked leafy green, yet Mother Nature blessed mustard greens with powerful detoxification properties that our bodies rely on to keep our body systems clean, strong and functioning at optimal levels. If we fail to give our body's detox system adequate nutritional support, yet continue to expose ourselves to toxins through poor lifestyle and dietary choices, we place our bodies at increased risk of toxin-related damage than can eventually increase our cell's risk of becoming cancerous. Mustard greens contain key phytonutrients called glucosinolates, which help activate detoxification enzymes and regulate their activity, thereby assisting our bodies in the constant purging of health-destroying free radicals, pathogens and toxic waste. For optimal detoxification benefits, incorporate mustard greens into your diet 3 times a week. Try them in vegetarian casserole dishes, stir fry's or even sautéed down with some fresh onion and garlic.

4. When it comes to heart health, romaine

lettuce is a fierce ally in maintaining cardiac balance. For starters, romaine is high in vitamin C and beta-carotene, a nutrient combination that effectively helps prevent the oxidation of cholesterol. This is important, because when cholesterol becomes oxidized, it becomes sticky and starts to adhere to lining of the arteries, causing dangerous plaque buildup. This can then lead to full-blown artery blockages, increasing one's risk of heart attack and stroke. Another important nutrient in romaine lettuce is folic acid. Folic acid is a B vitamin that is needed by the body to convert a damaging chemical called homocysteine into a benign substance that won't compromise cardiac health. If homocysteine is not converted, it can directly cause damage to blood vessels, thus greatly increasing the risk of heart attack and stroke. And, the fiber in romaine binds to bile salts in the digestive tract, signaling the body to produce more bile. This chemical reaction requires the breakdown of cholesterol for this process to happen, thereby reducing levels of bad cholesterol within the body. For these reasons, romaine lettuce should therefore be one of your base-lettuce choice for salads.

5. Kale contains a rich combination of anti-inflammatory and antioxidant properties, which make it a powerful defender and healer of oxidative stress and inflammation.

This is good news from those suffering from inflammatory conditions such as arthritis, gout, and rheumatism. Just one cup of fresh kale contains 10% omega-3 fatty acids and a megadose of vitamin K, which helps to knock down and prevent inflammatory responses in the body, thereby helping to relieve symptoms such as pain, swelling and stiffness. Oxidative stress within the body is caused by an imbalance of reactive oxygen and a biological system's ability to readily detoxify the offending matter, as well as an inhibited ability to repair damage to body tissues. Chronic oxidative stress due to poor lifestyle and dietary choices leads to the manifestation of illnesses, disease and infection, as well as hastens the aging-process. To slow down the aging process and reduce your risk of age-related disease and illness, make sure to include lots of fresh and cooked kale in your diet. Kale and mustard greens pair well together, and are delicious when sautéed down with garlic, onion, vegan bacon, salt and pepper.

6. Cancer prevention seems to be a standout health benefit of eating collard greens. The body's 3 major areas of defense against cancer are 1. The body's detoxification system 2. The body's antioxidant system 3. The body's inflammatory / anti-inflammatory system. Collard greens provide superior nutrient support of all 3 of these important systems, thus helping to

prevent cancer, as well as work to remedy and heal from it. Among all the types of cancer, prevention of the following types of cancer is most closely associated with the consumption of fresh collard greens: bladder cancer, colon cancer, breast cancer, lung cancer, prostate cancer and ovarian cancer. When you nutritional support the systems in your body that are responsible for maintaining homeostasis, you are naturally inclined to better health and well-being, as well as less likely to fall victim to ill-health, disease, rapid aging and obesity. Collard greens are one of those key vegetables that help provide you such nutritional support.

7. Mustard greens contain a vital nutrient combination, calcium, magnesium, folic acid and vitamin K, which makes mustard greens a necessary dark leafy vegetable to consume for good bone health. This nutrient combination helps stimulate new bone growth, maintain and improve bone density, and prevent the incidence of bone fractures. For those over the age of 40, and women in pre-menopausal and menopause years, maintaining good bone health is crucial, as the decline of female hormones increases a woman's risk of bone loss.

8. Swiss chard has excellent diuretic and laxative properties, making it a great remedy for the relief of constipation and water retention, as well as a natural detoxifier of

toxic waste from the body. If you're looking for a healthy way to shed excess weight, smooth out dimply cellulite, and clear your skin of acne, rashes and discolored blotchiness, Swiss chard can do all of that for you, and without the unwanted side effects of dangerous diet pills and crash diets. Swiss chard is also a very alkaline leafy green, which means it helps to reduce and remove acidic waste buildup in the body. Acidic waste is responsible for one's lack of ability to lose weight, as well as being a contributing factor to inflammatory conditions such as arthritis, gout and rheumatism, as well as auto-immune disorders. Swiss chard's ability to alkalize and detoxify your body, will help you shed stubborn fat stores, smooth out cellulite-prone areas of your skin, clear skin disruptions, balance mood, improve sleep and increase your body's ability to uptake nutrients from the foods you eat.

9. An effective remedy to rid bad breath is to regularly nosh on some fresh romaine lettuce. Romaine is rich in chlorophyll, a natural phytochemical found in plants that absorbs light from the sun and converts it into usable energy, and is responsible for making green plants, green in color. This chlorophyll found in romaine lettuce has potent cleansing and deodorizing properties, which make it highly beneficially to those trying to remedy bad breath. Additionally,

chlorophyll has anti-inflammatory and antibacterial properties that kill bad breath at its source. Suggested dosage of chlorophyll for the treatment of bad breath is 100mg – 300 mg daily. While you can certainly find a quality chlorophyll supplement, consuming chlorophyll from food sources is better absorbed by the body. A single large serving of romaine lettuce daily will help to freshen the breath in cases of mild halitosis, while in more severe cases, 2-3 servings of romaine lettuce a day is suggested until relief of symptoms is found, then a single serving daily for prevention is recommended.

10. Kale offers up a whopping 80 key vitamins and minerals in a single serving, and that's in addition to its incredibly high antioxidant quotient. This all-star lineup of nutrients is how kale optimally supports your immune system, fighting off pathogens and toxins and preventing them from taking hold within your body, to help keep you free of colds or flu. And, if you do happen to catch a cold or flu, drinking freshly juiced kale every day that you are sick will speed your recovery, reduce your symptoms and help to quickly bring your body back into a healthy balance. Kale and all dark, leafy green vegetables are truly nature's protection against illness and disease.

Melons:

Most melons have a similar structure to some squashes, in that they are thick fleshed and have a seed-filled midsection. In fact, both melons and squash belong to the same gourd family, which explains the similarities. While there are more melon varieties than you might think, in this remedy section I'll touch on the 3 most popular: honeydew, cantaloupe and watermelon. When purchasing a melon, regardless of which variety, it should feel heavy and be free of scars, tears and bruises. It's also best to purchase whole melons vs. ones that have been cut in half, as they will not be as fresh and will have already lost some of their nutrient value. Melons will also natural detach itself from the stem when it is ripe, and here's how you can tell if a melon is ripe when purchasing at the market. Check the stem button area of the melon. It should be yellowish in color, and have a fruity aroma coming from it. If it does not, it usually means the melon was cut before it was ripe. An uncut melon can be kept stored on your kitchen countertop for several days, or in the fridge for up to 2 weeks. Once cut, keep in the fridge and use within 2-3 days.

1. When it comes to keeping your skin wrinkle-free, taught and youthful looking, watermelon has got you covered on all

bases. For starters, the rind of watermelon is packed with vitamins, minerals and natural collagen-enhancing properties such as 'citrulline', and amino acid that aids the skin's healing and rejuvenation process. Additionally, lycopene, which is abundantly found in watermelon, has been proven to be twice as effective at protecting the skin from sun damage vs. beta-carotene. And, watermelon juice is rich in antioxidant and astringent properties, making it a great facial toner for those suffering from acne, rosacea, eczema and psoriasis. The easiest way to get all these amazing skin benefits, is to rub fresh watermelon rind across your freshly washed skin, and let air dry for 15 minutes before rinsing with cool water. If you commit to adding this into your normal skin care routine, you will be guaranteed wonderful results…and compliments.

2. Honeydew melon is a great fruit to add to your anti-aging diet, and is especially rich in vitamin C and the mineral potassium. Potassium is required by every cell in the body, and plays an important role in controlling blood pressure. Additionally, the combination of vitamin C and potassium boosts iron absorption in the body, providing support for those suffering from anemia and low energy. Honeydews are also loaded with the important nutrient folate. This is a crucial nutrient to consume regularly, as research has confirmed that

those who have low folate levels triple their risk of developing Alzheimer's disease. And, folate taken as a supplement doesn't have the same beneficial effects as it does when consumed through dietary sources. Suggested dosage for anti-aging benefits is to eat 3 cups of fresh honeydew weekly.

3. If you or someone you know smokes, eating cantaloupe on a very regular basis can protect you both from the dangers of smoking as well as the effects of secondhand smoke. Researchers have found severe vitamin A deficiency in both smokers and those exposed to secondhand smoke. They've also pinpointed a direct correlation between vitamin A deficiency and lung inflammation and emphysema, and that a common carcinogen in cigarette smoke 'benzo(a)pyrene' is at least one of the key causes of this vitamin A deficiency. A diet rich in vitamin A, which is found in abundance in fresh cantaloupe, can significantly counter this effect and reduce one's incidence of emphysema in both smokers and non-smokers exposed to secondhand smoke.

4. Watermelon is extremely cleansing to the entire body, including the colon, heart, skin, liver, bladder, stomach and kidneys. Watermelon has been used extensively for centuries as a natural remedy in those suffering from kidney stones, frequent UTI's

(urinary tract infections and other urological imbalances. Too much caffeine, protein, alcohol and fast foods put a major strain on the kidneys, leading to their impaired ability to breakdown and flush toxic waste from the body. This can then lead to kidney stones, bladder and kidney infections and even kidney failure. In addition to cleaning up your overall diet and lifestyle, you can benefit from regularly drinking fresh watermelon juice daily, or even doing a full 1-3 day watermelon cleanse. Drinking fresh watermelon juice stimulates the clearing of toxic waste, including uric acid from the body, reducing the strain on the body's filtering systems, including the kidneys, liver, bladder and skin. You can either drink 1 glass daily in the morning on an empty stomach, or do a full cleanse, which means you'll be consuming fresh watermelon juice 3 times a day along with plenty of fresh water. Watermelon juice is also a blood tonic, and therefore very rejuvenating, so you won't feel fatigued. If you already have kidney disease and are on doctor's protocol, do not do this cleanse without first consulting with your doctor.

5. For some readers, you love honeydew melon, cantaloupe and watermelon, but you seem to get an upset stomach after eating them. The reason may be in your food consumption timing. Any type of melon should always be eating by itself and with a

short time delay before consuming any additional food or beverage. Eating melons this way will allow you to enjoy both their taste as well as their health benefits, but without digestive upset. By the way, eating on an empty stomach means first thing in the morning, or 4 hours after your last bite of food. After eating melon, wait 30 minutes before consuming any additional food or drink. That being said, all 3 of these melon varieties are filled with healthy fruit fiber, which gently scrub your digestive tract of accumulated waste, thereby relieving constipation, excess gas, bloating and weight gain due to toxic waste buildup within the body.

6. To prevent the ravages of summer weather, including heat, sun, chlorine and wind from causing havoc on your hair, try this easy to make pre-shampoo hair treatment using fresh cantaloupe. In a blender, combine 1 large, ripe banana (diced), ½ of a ripe avocado (diced), approximately ¼ of a small cantaloupe (diced) and 2 tablespoons plain yogurt, and puree until smooth. First brush out hair to remove any styling product residue, and liberally coat your hair, paying particular attention to the ends, with the cantaloupe hair mask. Cover with a shower cap, and let sit for 15-30 minutes before washing out and shampooing as normal. The nutrients and antioxidants in the cantaloupe help to protect and moisturize your hair

cuticles, nourish your scalp, and prevent breakage. You can use this hair mask 1-3 times weekly, and is safe to use for colored hair and bleached hair. For longer hair, just double the recipe.

7. For a super-fast clearing of acne, honeydew melon can help you see clear skin in just days. Eating 1-2 servings of fresh honeydew daily, along with swiping the inside rind across freshly washed skin, helps provide the skin with all the necessary nutrients it needs to balance oil production in your skin pores, gently exfoliate dead skin and toxic residue off the surface of your skin, and aids in balancing hormone responses within your body that may be out of balance and thereby perhaps being a contributing factor to your acne and blackhead breakouts. When using the rind as a toner mask, first wash face with a pH balanced, gentle cleanser. Allow face to air dry, then moisten a cotton ball with hydrogen peroxide and give your entire face area a good swipe. Again, allow skin to air dry, then swipe your face with the inside rind part of a piece of honeydew melon. Allow the residue to sit for 15-30 minutes, and then rinse off with cool water. Do this daily, for quick results, and then as needed for clear skin maintenance.

8. Consuming fresh watermelon when you are out in the hot summer heat, or after exercise, is a much healthier alternative than

chemical-laden sports drinks. Fresh watermelon can replace those electrolytes lost during physical activity and sweating, helping to quickly bring your body's mineral content back into balance and prevent muscle cramping and brain fog. Eating watermelon also has a natural cooling effect, helping to reduce the heat discomfort of the sun, as well as provide your body with natural defenses against the harmful effects of sun radiation. And, since watermelon's content is 90-95% water, it is an excellent dietary source of hydration.

9. Studies have shown that the average person consumes 3 pounds worth of food a day. That's a lot more food than many of us realize. One of the premises behind volumetric eating is to eat foods dense in water, natural fiber and nutrients, which actually help to keep you feeling fuller and satiated better than dense, fried, fatty food options. And, when it comes to managing our hunger, eating foods high in water such as melons, actually does a better job at appetite control vs. consuming solid food along with a glass of water. Eating lots of fresh melons, such as honeydew, cantaloupe and watermelon, all help you to lose weight easily while still maintaining your energy, while flooding your body will enormous amounts of usable nutrients, including vitamins, minerals and amino acids. If you'd like to eat melon for weight loss, consume

2-3 cups of fresh melon each morning on an empty stomach. Eat a healthy lunch and dinner, and consume lots of fresh water and herbal teas. Choose whichever melon variety you like best, and change them up as your palate dictates, but AVOID mixing melon varieties together at the same time, as this can lead to potential digestive upset.

10. Got a hangover? Drinking lots of water after a night of drinking helps, but drinking fresh watermelon juice helps even better. Watermelon's diuretic effects help to move toxic alcohol by-products out of your system faster, while the minerals in the watermelon help to restore electrolyte balance. The high antioxidant properties in watermelon also work to neutralize free radical activity caused by drinking alcohol, thereby preventing alcohol-induced free radical damage to the body. For best results, drink 1 glass of fresh watermelon juice (or eat 2 cups of cubed watermelon) every few hours, with nothing else other than water. You can 'spice up' your watermelon juice by adding some fresh grated ginger or a squeeze of fresh lime juice (both of which provide additional detoxification benefits), but do not add anything else.

Mushrooms:

The 'king' of mushrooms is probably the Reishi variety, but there are many more to choose from, including cremini, button, shiitake, Portobello and oyster, and they all provide lots of health benefits. When purchasing mushrooms, only pick-up what you will use within 5 days, as they are highly perishable. Choose mushrooms that are firm, and free of bruising. You don't want any that look like they have a slimy film on them, which is more prevalent in prepackaged mushroom vs. mushrooms bought in bulk. Mushrooms should be stored either in a brown paper bag or open container in the fridge, and never in plastic, as this causes them to 'sweat' and will hasten their disintegration. Another note on purchasing mushrooms is that you should ALWAYS buy organic. Mushrooms are incredibly porous, meaning they act like little sponges, and readily soak in toxic pesticides and herbicides typically used in commercial farming. You cannot wash this off of mushrooms, or any other fruit or veggie for that matter, so if you can't buy organic with all your veggies, at least make sure to buy organic mushrooms to avoid ingesting these dangerous chemicals.

1. Mushrooms are a dieter's dream. They are an excellent substitute for meat in dishes, are virtually fat free, contain no artery-clogging

cholesterol, and have a scant 15-25 calories per cup, depending on the variety. They are very filling, and their combination low-carb and high-fiber content help keep blood sugar levels stable. Keeping blood sugar levels stable is a key factor in fending off food cravings, food binges and mood disturbances caused by erratic swings in blood sugar. Unlike most vegetables, mushrooms contain 2 important B vitamins – niacin and riboflavin, in addition to vitamins C, D, B6 and B12, making mushrooms a nutritional powerhouse. And, when it comes to shaving off calories….swapping just one 4 ounce serving of mushrooms in place of 4 ounces of meat, once a week for a year, could save you more than 18,000 calories and 3,000 grams of saturated fat. AND, that's just by swapping out once a week. Imagine how many more calories you could save by doing this multiple times a week. Mushrooms are so versatile, and easy to prepare in so many dishes, there's no excuse for not using them, especially when it comes to adding them to a healthy weight loss menu.

2. A not-so-well known mushroom variety here in the west, yet highly prized in Asian cultures, is a mushroom species called tremella. It is used in Traditional Chinese Medicine for a multitude of purposes, and is also revered by Asian women for its superior anti-aging properties for skin and

body. For starters, consuming tremella mushrooms (or the extract) on a regular basis, seems to be a natural weight loss aid, as it is an appetite suppressant, digestive regulatory and whole body detoxifier. And, when it comes to skin care, there is a reason why this mushroom species is so coveted by Asian women. A unique polysaccharide found in tremella mushrooms, gives it the ability to hold up to 500 times its weight in water, which is far, far more than those hyaluronic acid facial topical treatments can even come close to. Why is this important? Hyaluronic acid is a natural-occurring carbohydrate compound that is found in various parts of the body, especially in skin tissue. It helps the skin to retain moisture, and is the reason why this ingredient is often found in anti-aging skin care products. It's highly effective. In research studies, when tremella mushroom was taken both internally, as well as applied topically, participants noticed a very visible difference in their skin within the first 30 days. Their face was fuller and more youthful looking, and their fine lines and wrinkles were smoothed out due to their skin's new ability to absorb and retain moisture. To find tremella mushrooms as well as topical preparations using an extract of the mushroom, you'll need to find an Asian market near you, or search for a reputable vendor online.

3. Probably one of the most popular uses for medicinal mushrooms is for an overall anti-aging, immune system tonic, and is commonly used for this purpose in Traditional Chinese medicine. In Asian cultures, medicinal mushrooms are consumed regularly, for the maintenance of one's health and well-being, and is especially effective at preventing the incidence of colds, flu, infection and other illness. Here is just a sampling of the benefits these medicinal mushrooms offer. Reishi mushroom users were found to have 'acute spikes' of antioxidant properties in their blood stream, which is crucial to neutralizing and preventing harmful free radical damage, as well as providing extreme boosts to one's immune system function. Gypsy mushroom is shown to have specific defending properties against flu viruses. Cordyceps mushroom increases white blood cell activity when alerted to the presence of a pathogen, which then stimulates the immune system response and effectively killing the offending microorganisms. Maitake mushrooms have been shown to stimulate the production of a certain protein needed by the immune system, to defend the body against colds, flu and infection. To get these amazing medicinal mushroom benefits, just visit your local health food store, and start picking up some of these mushroom varieties to add to

your diet. You can also look for medicinal mushroom extracts, which are offered in both single mushroom and multiple mushroom combinations.

4. Cordyceps mushroom is a powerful aid to both men and women who are suffering for low libido and sexual arousal disruptions. Cordyceps is a vasodilator, meaning it expands blood vessels and improves circulation, which means more blood and oxygen to the genital area for both men and women. And, for men, cordyceps influences the release of testosterone, increases the rigidity of erections, and helps increase sperm's motility. Cordyceps is really a great overall aphrodisiac for both men and women. And, sheep herders in Tibet even feed it to their flock to increase desire, sexual activity and reproduction. Many professional athletes around the world take cordyceps for stamina, strength, speed of recovery and all-around heightened athletic ability, so you know it must obviously work.

5. Shitake is the second most cultivated mushroom variety in the world, and is prized for its rich anti-viral, anti-tumor, anti-fungal properties for the natural prevention and treatment of cancer and AIDS patients. Shitake mushrooms naturally produce interferon, which is considered to be the reason behind its anti-viral results. Shitake mushrooms also contain a compound called

'lentinan', which helps it to avert damage to chromosomes that may otherwise be initiated by anti-cancer drugs. In Japan, lentinan is extracted from shitake mushrooms and used as an official drug for cancer patients. It is even given to patients prior to radiation treatments, to help fend off unwanted side effects, and keep the patient's immune system strong. A diet rich in shitake mushrooms can improve one's immune system function, as well as build an on-going defense against invading organisms.

Nuts:

Most nuts contain mono-unsaturated fats, which is the healthy kind your body requires for optimal function. And, most nuts are so nutritious that you only need to consume 1-2 handfuls a day. A 'serving' of nuts is ½ ounce. You ideally only want to purchase and consume raw nuts, vs. pasteurized ones, and only purchase what you'll consume within 2 weeks (or 1 month if stored in fridge), as they are highly perishable. Buying raw nuts from the bulk bins at natural health food markets is a good choice, since they tend to move pretty quickly, reducing the likelihood that you'll be purchasing rancid nuts. The best way to store raw nuts is in a tightly sealed container in the fridge, or second best, in a cool dark pantry. To extend their freshness even longer, you can store them in the freezer in a tightly sealed baggie for up to 3 months. This is especially helpful during the holidays when you might be using extra amounts of them.

1. Did you know that almonds have been long used and prized as an aphrodisiac? Eating almonds stimulates the flow of blood to the genital region and increases the flow of sexual fluids in both men and women. And, while their scent is subtle, science has shown that almond's aroma is stimulating to both females and males. In many cultures, this is also one of the reasons why you see sugared almonds on the wedding party and guests tables at weddings. It is symbolic of sex and fertility. So, the next time you want to kick up your sex drive during a romantic evening with your partner, skip the cake for dessert and have some fresh, raw almonds instead.

2. Coconut water is the clear liquid inside of a fresh coconut, and coconut milk is the combination of this water along with the white pulp meat inside the coconut. Both are highly nutritious and unless you are allergic to coconuts, I'd recommend adding coconut water, milk, cream and pulp meat in your diet, as well as for natural remedies. For topical skin preparations, coconut water or milk (or even unrefined, virgin coconut oil)

can be brushed onto the skin in a thin layer, to help heal minor burns, ringworm, eczema, poison ivy and other skin inflammations. Coconut's antimicrobial, antifungal, anti-inflammatory and antiseptic properties quickly go to work, to mend and heal inflammatory conditions, while the rare fat molecules in coconut's medium chain fatty acids actually annihilate a wide range of skin disease-causing toxins and organisms. For severe skin disruption such as skin ulcers and boils, mix fresh coconut water or milk with just enough rice flour to make a paste, and spread evenly over affected skin areas. Rinse and apply a fresh coconut plaster twice a day, until condition improves.

3. For those who suffer from either Type I herpes or Type II herpes, consuming pine nuts on a regular basis can help reduce your incidence of outbreak, lessen the severity of your symptoms and speed healing to reduce outbreak time. Pine nuts are very rich in the amino acid lysine, which is scientifically proven to reduce herpes outbreaks and symptoms. So, in addition to reducing your food intake of foods rich in L-arginine, add in a serving (1/2 ounce) of pine nuts to your daily diet. They have a mild, creamy flavor and blend well with salads, pasta dishes, vegetables and casseroles.

4. How would you like to lose up to 40 pounds

a year, without changing your diet or exercise routine? Sounds like a dream right? Well, by consuming coconut oil daily, you can do just that. Coconut oil is made up of MCT (medium change triglycerides), which when consumed, head straight to your liver where it is immediately burned to produce energy. This metabolic process revs up your rate of metabolism, and in fact, a single serving of coconut oil in place of other cooking oils or fats, can raise your metabolic rate for up to 24 hours. Unless you're allergic to coconuts, there are no side effects, just increased energy and decreased weight. And, if you suffer from weight gain due to a sluggish thyroid, coconut oil supports and encourages your thyroid to produce thyroid hormones, thus helping to bring your thyroid function into a healthier balance. Again, no side effects, just an increase in thyroid activity and a decrease in weight. For weight loss and thyroid balancing benefits, you ideally want to be consuming 3 tablespoons of virgin, unrefined coconut oil on a daily basis. You can easily get your daily quota of coconut oil by taking a spoonful before meals, mixing it in with a smoothie, or use it in place of your other cooking oils. However you consume coconut oil, make sure to ONLY consume virgin, unrefined coconut oil. Never use refined coconut oil internally or externally.

5. Instead of turning to potentially dangerous chemical peels to keep your skin smooth, bright and wrinkle-free, try this do-it-yourself facial scrub using ground almonds. In a coffee or spice grinder, grind up 8-10 raw almonds. Transfer into a small mixing bowl, and add in 2 teaspoons of cream and 2 teaspoons of raw honey, stirring until well blended. After washing face, neck and décolletage area with a gentle soap-free cleanser, first allow skin to air dry, then using circular motions, gently massage in the almond skin scrub. Massage for a full 2 minutes, then leave the residue sit on the skin for an additional 10-15 minutes. Rinse with cool water, and apply a mineral oil-free moisturizer. The almonds will naturally exfoliate dead skin cells and debris, while at the same time stimulating the growth of new skin cells. As we age, natural skin cell turnover becomes slower and slower, so we can help things along with natural skin scrubs. The lactic acid in the cream will also help to exfoliate, while the fatty acids will encourage moisture retention in the skin. The raw honey is brimming with antibacterial, antiseptic and antioxidant properties, which help to kill off bacteria, while at the same time infusing the skin with vital nutrients and moisture retention abilities. Use this facial scrub 1-2 times a week, as part of your anti-aging skin care routine.

6. For those looking to reduce the urge to drink alcohol and tone and heal their liver, try this non-alcoholic nut cocktail using raw macadamias. In a blender, combine 5-7 raw macadamia nuts, 3 very ripe tomatoes (diced), ½ teaspoon of freshly-squeezed lemon juice, a pinch of cayenne pepper powder, and a teaspoon of freshly grated ginger root. Blend until all ingredients are well blended and smooth. Transfer into a serving glass, stir in any optional salt and pepper as desired and enjoy. The macadamia nuts and other ingredients in this cocktail help to squash the urge to drink alcohol, and equally as important, also help to rejuvenate the liver.

7. A unique, yet highly effective remedy for fungal infections of the fingernails or toenails, as well as jock itch, is an old Ayurvedic recipe using sun dried coconut. To make this remedy, crack open a ripe coconut in half (save the water to drink), and allow the halved coconut shells to sit in the sun for a week. After a week's worth of sun drying, smash up the coconut shells with a hammer. Gather up all the fragments and soak them in 1 quart of vodka for 10-14 days, shaking the solution twice a day. After 10-14 days, strain the solution and keep in an airtight container out of direct light. For jock itch, after bathing, saturate a cotton ball with the coconut elixir and swab the groin area fully. Allow to air dry before dressing.

For finger or toenail fungal infections, add a couple tablespoons of coconut elixir into a bowl or foot bath, along with enough hot water to cover hands or feet, and soak for 30 minutes. Alternately, you can also swab the affected fingers or toenails with a saturated cotton ball, and allow to air dry. This remedy typically works relatively quickly, if you use it regularly.

8. Another unique skin remedy using nuts, is for the healing of skin rashes, age spots, acne, ringworm and warts, and requires the use of either green or immature black walnuts. The remedy is extremely simple. Just cut a couple incisions into the outer shell of the walnut, and rub the juice onto the affected skin area. At first there might be a slight stinging sensation, but it should disappear in short order. You also might experience some skin staining from the walnut juice, but this will wear off and is not permanent. The walnuts contain healing anti-inflammatory properties, as well as sterols, tannins and iodine, which all contribute to the fast healing of these various skin conditions.

9. If you live in an area where there are lots of oak trees, here is a fantastic burn remedy used by the Iroquois Indian tribe using acorns. Gather up a couple large handfuls of fresh acorns. Place them in a large Ziploc bag, and smash them up using a hammer or

rolling pin. Dump the crushed acorn pieces into a medium sized saucepan filled with water, and bring to a boil for 1 minute. Immediately reduce heat, and simmer until liquid has reduced to half the original amount (2-3 hours). This releases and infuses the water with the healing tannic acids from the acorns. Strain and transfer into a sealable, glass container. Solution will keep fresh in the fridge for several months. Anytime you, or someone in your family gets a minor burn, skin scrape, skin rash or but bite, swab the affected area with the acorn solution and allow to air dry. Wait at least 6 hours before washing off and reapplying as needed.

10. For cases of bad breath and minor toothache, filberts can help neutralize offending mouth odor, as well as relieve the throbbing of a toothache. For cases of bad breath, simply chewing slowly on a filbert nut for several minutes or more, actually neutralizes and absorbs the bacteria responsible for causing the offensive odor, vs. just masking the odor the way breath mints, gum and mouthwashes do. For cases of minor toothache, while you're waiting to see your dentist, grind a couple filbert nuts up in a coffee or spice grinder until the consistency if of a fine powder. Mix it with a dollop of raw honey (never use processed honey) and apply the filbert mixture onto the affected tooth area, to relieve painful throbbing.

Olives:

Olive are technically a fruit, are available year round, and can be purchased fresh in the produce or deli section of your market, as well as in cans and jars. Once purchased, you always want to keep your olive submerged in the brine liquid it comes in. If purchased in a plastic or glass container, you can keep in the fridge for a couple months. If you've purchased olives in a can, if you don't use them all at one time, transfer the remaining olive, along with the brine juice, into a glass or plastic container and store in the fridge. Olives are jammed-packed with flavor, phytonutrients, healthy fats and health and beauty benefits.

1. If you suffer from minor allergies, you might be interested in knowing that olives have long been used in herbal medicine practices for the treatment of inflammatory conditions, including allergy-related conditions. Compounds found in olives have been shown to have antihistamine properties. These compounds work by blocking special histamine receptors, and lessening a cell's histamine response. This is important, because histamine is a molecule that can get over-produced in allergy-related conditions. For this reason, fresh olives have been long prescribed by herbal practitioners

in an anti-allergenic diet. Additionally, olives are very rich in antioxidant properties, which effectively help to neutralize cellular damage caused by free radicals, including inflammation, adding another layer of protection against allergens as well as reducing the body's responses to them.

2. For those who are looking to tighten up loose, sagging skin due to age or weight loss, here is a coveted holistic spa recipe you can make at home. In a blender, combine 2 eggs yolks (reserve the whites) with ½ cup of fresh olives, and puree until mixture is smooth and creamy in texture. After first washing skin and allowing to air dry, brush the olive-yolk mixture evenly across the areas of skin you wish to tighten (skin, neck, décolletage, stomach), and allow mixture to sit for 10 minutes. While mixture is drying, beat the reserved egg whites until they form stiff peaks, and after 10 minutes, brush the beaten egg whites over the top, and let the entire 2 layer mask sit for 1 hour. Rinse with cool water and apply a mineral oil-free moisturizer. Do this 3 times a week and really watch how your skin starts to lift and tighten.

3. One of my grandmother's favorite remedies for earaches was garlic infused olive oil. The garlic-olive oil combination lends antiseptic, antibacterial and anti-inflammatory properties that help fight off infection and

reduce inflammation, bringing quick relief from swelling, pain and pressure. To make this remedy, slice a fresh clove of garlic and let it soak in 2 ounces of olive oil for 1 hour, to allow the garlic properties to be infused into the oil. After an hour, strain out the garlic and gently warm the garlic olive oil in a small saucepan slightly, until just lukewarm in temperature. Using a dropper, slowly squeeze or drip 5 drops into the affected ear, while keeping the head tilted to the opposite side. GENTLY rub the earlobe afterwards for about 30 seconds, and wipe off any excess dripping oil. Massaging the earlobe will help allow the oil to get deeper into the ear canal, so it can come in contact with the inflamed area where it is needed. Try to lay still for at least 30 minutes, and if both ears are affected, wait 15 minutes before apply the oil to the other ear. This remedy is for mild earaches and possible mild ear infections only. If your condition doesn't change for the better, or if symptoms worsen, seek medical attention.

4. If your baby or grand-baby is having teething discomfort, rubbing a thin layer of olive oil directly onto their gums will help bring almost immediate relief. Olive oil's anti-inflammatory properties will quickly go to work to reduce swelling and pressure, while also helping to knock down pain and discomfort much like a NSAID (non-steroidal anti-inflammatory drug) such as

aspirin or ibuprofen does, without any unwanted side effects. It's safe for baby, but only apply the oil to baby's gums when you are awake and able to monitor the child.

5. Dandruff can make a mess of both your clothes and your personal life as well. Here is a very effective home remedy that will help rid your scalp of all those embarrassing flakes, while at the same time actually go to work to heal the source of the problem. In a small bowl, whisk together equal parts of olive oil and apple cider vinegar (do not use white vinegar). Before going to bed, brush your hair to rid styling product residue and tangles, and massage the olive oil and vinegar mixture into all areas of your scalp using the pads of your fingers for at least 3 minutes. You really want to coat the scalp. The olive oil is naturally clarifying, so it will help loosen away debris that might be clogging the hair follicles. The vinegar can then go to work to further dissolve away any follicle-clogging debris, while at the same time nourish your scalp with minerals and enzymes needed for healthy scalp and hair. I cannot emphasize enough, only use apple cider vinegar with the 'mother' enzyme in it, along with extra-virgin olive oil for this remedy. Once you've applied the oil mixture to the scalp, cover with a shower cap, and keep on head overnight. You might want to also put an old towel down on your pillow to protect it from drips. In the morning, first do

a water only rinse, then add 1 teaspoon of baking soda to your shampoo to wash your hair as normal. The baking soda will help to remove all the loosened skin cells and other debris that the oil mixture removed during the night. For severe cases of dandruff, do this every other day until symptoms improve, then once a week or more as needed for prevention.

Peaches:

Peaches are a sweet summer fruit, and unfortunately, are not available everywhere. The many varieties of peaches means that they come in different colors, but don't let color be your guide to ripeness. Any peach that has green around its stem base, means that it was picked prematurely and you should avoid buying those. Peaches are actually quite fragile, so don't start pushing your finger into to them to judge ripeness. In addition to avoiding peaches with bruises, tears and wrinkled skin, pick up the peach in your hand to judge its firmness and texture. You don't want it too soft or too firm. Additionally, the peach should be giving off a distinct aroma of peach. Ripe peaches will last 1-2 days at room temperature, or up to 5 days in the crisper drawer in your fridge. They also freeze well, so if you wish to keep them for holiday baking, slice up the peaches into segments and store in a freezer-proof plastic bag for up to 6 months.

1. Peaches are excellent for digestive health, and are easily assimilated by even the most sensitive of stomachs. The natural fruit fiber in peach, gives it gentle and effective laxative benefits, while the alkaline juices stimulate the digestive fluids needed to properly breakdown food and utilize its nutrients. Peaches are even well tolerated amongst those who suffer from stomach ulcers and inflammation of the bowels. For severe digestive system cases, peaches are better tolerated cooked vs. raw. For relief from constipation, or just to keep the bowels regular, eat a fresh peach 3 hours before bed. In addition to being highly cleansing to the digestive tract, peaches are also very cleansing for the kidneys.

2. Peaches are also incredibly beneficial for eye health, and preventing age-related eye conditions. The compounds lutein and zeaxanthin found in peaches, help protect eyes from scorching heat, as well as protect against age-related conditions such as cataracts and macular degeneration. The antioxidants in peaches help neutralize free radical damage, which left unchecked, would lead to oxidative stress to eye tissue. Additional, the vitamin A content in peaches also helps strengthen night vision. For

protection from age-related eye conditions, as well as protection against the ravages of summer's heat and often intense sunrays, make sure to eat lots of fresh summer peaches while they're in season.

3. For a no-nonsense, yet effective way to brighten and tighten your skin, here's a way you can have a peaches and cream complexion just by using the skin of a peach. Very gently, peel the skin off a ripe peach. After washing skin, and allow it to air dry, again, very gently (you don't want to tear the peel) rub the inside of the peach peel all across your face, neck and décolletage area. Ideally, you want to do this before bed, and leave the peach residue on your skin overnight, before rinsing off with cool water in the morning. The inside of the peel has natural astringent properties which help pull debris from your skin pores, while at the same time shrinking and tightening the appearance of the pores. The phytonutrients and antioxidants in the peach peel go to work to nourish skin cells, stimulate skin cell turnover and protect against free radical damage which could otherwise lead to fine lines, wrinkles, sagging and crepey skin. If you spend a lot of time outdoors in the summer, this peach peel remedy can help keep your skin young and healthy looking, giving you that peaches-and-cream glow.

4. Anemia is a condition in which the body has

a decrease in the number of red blood cells, which often leads to extreme fatigue and weakness. Oxygen is transported throughout the body via red blood cells, and when red blood cells are low, oxygen levels are lower, and energy is lower. And, when your body is low in iron, it can lead to iron-deficiency anemia. Iron supplements can be very risky to take, and should never be taken without the direction of your doctor. Taking an excess of iron supplements can lead to liver damage, and is serious business. Instead, replacing low iron stores is best done through nutritional sources, and peaches happen to be a healthy, iron-rich fruit. Additionally, the alkalizing juice in peaches is very toning to the blood, heart and brain, which also aids in increasing oxygen and energy levels within the body. Eating a fresh peach daily for the treatment and prevention of iron-deficiency anemia is a much healthier and safer way to go.

5. If you are suffering from a scratchy sore throat, cough or laryngitis (inflammation of the vocal chords), try this brandied peach recipe which has been handed down for generations in many an Italian family, for quick effective relief. Fill a 1 or 2 quart container ¾ of the way full with sliced or diced fresh peaches. Next, add in 2 cups of brandy and 1 cup of sugar and stir. If this doesn't cover all the peaches, add in some more brandy and sugar, until the solution

covers the fruit. Cover container (easiest to make in a 2 quart pitcher) and place in the fridge. Refrigerate for at least 2 weeks before using, making sure to stir or shake the container once a day. Then, when you have a sore throat, cough, etc., just spoon out 1 tablespoon of brandied peach dices and consume along with a couple swallows of warm water (not cold). This will calm throat spasms, heal inflamed throat and mouth tissues and kill off pathogens. Note: This remedy is for adults only, and should not be given to children due to the alcohol content. Mixture will keep fresh in the fridge for at least a couple months.

Peppers:

Peppers are fruits and broadly divided into two categories, sweet peppers and hot peppers. Both varieties are loaded with flavor and health benefits, and are easy to cook with, making them a favorite vegetable in the kitchen. Sweet peppers are typically known as bell peppers, and come in green, red, orange and yellow varieties. When purchasing sweet peppers, regardless of which color you're choosing, it should feel firm and heavy in your hand and be free of bruising, soft spots and skin wrinkling. Sweet peppers store best in a plastic bag in your fridge, and typically stay fresh for about a week. For whatever reason, green peppers seem to last a little longer than its red, orange and yellow cousins. In very general terms, hot peppers are commonly known as chili peppers, but there is quite a variety amongst them, including in their 'heat' factor. Common hot peppers include jalapeno pepper, Serrano pepper, Tai chili pepper, Fresno pepper, Habanero pepper, cherry pepper, banana pepper, Chili Verde pepper and cayenne pepper. Using just a few of these as examples, here is a range of these peppers 'heat' factor, starting from the mildest to the hottest. Bell – Cherry – Poblano – Jalapeno – Serrano – Cayenne – Tai – Habanero. Regardless of pepper species, much of their heat is contained in their seeds. Avoid touching your face, especially your eyes when handling hot peppers. To store hot peppers, rinse them in cool water, dry thoroughly, and place in a sealed plastic bag in the crisper drawer of your fridge. They will keep fresh for up to a week.

1. Red bell peppers have just the right phytonutrient, flavonoid and antioxidant combination to make them a perfect dietary protector against heart disease and stroke, two of the most prevalent age-related health concerns. The capsaicin and flavonoids in red bell peppers works to keep blood vessels dilated, thus helping to keep blood pressure down and reducing the risk of a dangerous blood clot. This compound combination also works to help lower levels of bad cholesterol

by breaking up oxidized cholesterol deposits from the artery walls, so that the body can then expel them. When allowed to fully ripen, red bell peppers are very high in vitamin C, a vital antioxidant our bodies require to neutralize and protect against free radical damage that can lead to heart and blood vessel damage. For these heart health benefits, red bell peppers are best consumed raw, since long cooking times destroys much of their nutritional value. The second best eating option would be to steam or stir fry them, both of which only require short cooking times.

2. To help stop bleeding from a cut, scrape or other injury, using either fresh cut cayenne peppers or cayenne powder, will help stop bleeding and start clotting blood in just minutes. Used internally or externally, cayenne immediately goes to work equalizing blood pressure throughout the whole body, thus keeping focalized pressure away from the hemorrhaging wound so that the blood will clot naturally. To use a fresh cayenne pepper, simply make a slice lengthwise but not all the way through, and filet open the pepper. Do not wash or brush away the seeds, as you want them intact. Place the filleted pepper directly onto the wound, and gently hold in place until bleeding starts to subside. If you don't have fresh cayenne peppers, but have cayenne powder, you can sprinkle a pinch or two

directly onto the wound, and let it stay in place until well after the bleeding stops. For even faster and more substantial bleeding relief, you can put a very tiny pinch of cayenne powder into a glass of warm water, and drink back quickly as soon as you can after the injury. The warm water will open up the cells and the cayenne will go to work in less than 1 minutes normalizing blood pressure. Drinking cayenne this way on an empty stomach will cause some minor discomfort, but if you really need to stop the bleeding, it's worth the temporary inconvenience. If you've recently eaten, you should notice no stinging or discomfort whatsoever, unless you go overboard with the amount of cayenne you use. And, if the bleeding is significant enough to require sutures or other medical attention, immediately head to the hospital.

3. Consuming any of the hot pepper varieties is very supporting to one's sexual well-being, and heightens the experience for both men and women alike. The capsaicin in all hot peppers is a vasodilator, and increases blood and oxygen circulation to the genital region, engorging the clitoris in women and the penis in men. Erections for men may also be harder and increase in duration. To enjoy these sexual health benefits, try enjoying a romantic dinner over spicy Mexican or Asian food. Or, here's another way you can increase the mood. After dinner, order up

some fresh, hot coffee and sprinkle a tiny pinch of cayenne powder into the coffee, stir and drink. You can certainly add cream, sugar or liquor as well. The caffeine in the coffee will actually heighten cayenne's benefits even further, and since you've buffered your stomach with food from dinner, you should only notice a 'warming' sensation, and not any burning or stinging. You'll feel the results quickly, and in my personal opinion, this pepper libido enhancer works better than any other natural aphrodisiac.

4. One of the most commonly used peppers by herbal medicine practitioners for the relief of pain and inflammation, is cayenne pepper. Even western medicine has been adding capsaicin, one of cayenne peppers main compounds, into everything from cayenne capsules, to cayenne ointments, sprays and even cayenne pain patches. The reason why is, it works. Once cayenne is ingested (or even applied topically), it immediately binds to various nerve receptors in the body, and interrupts the flow of pain signals to the brain. As the capsaicin is being distributed throughout the body, you might initially notice a slight increase in pain, but within minutes as the pain signals are no longer able to reach the brain, it will quickly disappear completely or bring you a significant reduction to your discomfort. Additionally, cayenne peppers (as well as

other hot peppers) naturally boost the body's production of endorphins, which act as natural painkillers in the body, thus providing another level of relief from your pain and inflammation. To get these natural pain relief benefits, you can either eat lots of fresh hot peppers in your daily diet, or for convenience purposes, take cayenne powder in supplement form from a reputable vendor.

5. Both sweet and hot peppers make food choices for a healthy weight loss plan. Peppers are very low in calories, have a high water content, and are a surprising source of dietary fiber. This combination means that you're body has to work hard and longer to digest peppers, helping you feel full faster and staying full longer. And, because their loaded with phytonutrients, they naturally squash food cravings for unhealthy food choices. For weight loss benefits, it is best to consume both sweet and hot peppers raw as often as possible, for maximum benefits. And, the capsaicin compound found in peppers naturally stokes your metabolic rate so that you burn fat and calories faster for up to 24 hours after consuming. Eat some peppers on a daily basis, and you'll keep your metabolism on fire.

Plums and Prunes:

There are over 125 varieties of plums, and most of them are grown for drying into prunes. Fresh plums are typically available mid-summer to mid-autumn, and are a bit on the fragile side. When purchasing fresh plums, be sure to only choose plums that do not have any skin tears, bruising, soft spots or wrinkling. Color should be even, and the overall texture should be firm but give slightly when given a gentle squeeze. Plums are best stored at room temperature and used within 2 days. They will keep fresh in the fridge for up to a week, but their quality is diminished when refrigerated. When purchasing prunes, especially those bought from the bulk bin at your natural food market, they should be plump, shiny, relatively soft and free of mold. Prunes are best stored in an airtight container, and kept in a cool, dry cabinet or pantry, where they will keep fresh for several months.

1. Age we age, our digestive system doesn't function as smoothly as it did in our youth, so making sure we support digestive health with good dietary choices is important. And, our bodies respond much better to food sources of fiber vs. harsh fiber supplements that can cause even more digestive upset. Just one of the reasons why that is the case, is that by consuming foods rich in natural

fiber, you are constantly supplying your body with small, yet regular doses of natural-occurring fiber. This is well tolerated by the body, vs. dumping huge amounts of fiber-laden supplements or drinks into the body, which actually ends up clogging the digestive system even more, further aggravating constipation, excess gas and bloating. The fiber content found in plums and prunes isn't the only reason why it makes a good laxative and digestive system regulator. Plums, and especially prunes, are high in naturally-occurring sugars, which once inside the digestive tract, attract and bind water into the central cavity, helping to soften stools and expedite their release. To relieve a current bout of constipation, drink 8 ounces of cold water, followed by 4-5 large prunes 1 hour later. If relief is not had within 4 hours, eat another 4-5 prunes. For prevention of constipation, and maintenance of digestive health, eat 3 prunes nightly, 3 hours before bedtime.

2. Said to be a secret skin care application amongst the beautiful Japanese Geishas, here is a simple plum mask you can make at home to both brighten and tighten your skin. In a blender, combine 2 plums (diced with skin left on) and 2 egg whites, and puree until mixture is well combined, about 1-2 minutes. After first washing face and allowing it to air dry, brush the plum mask evenly across face, neck and décolletage

area, and allow it set for 30 minutes. Rinse off with cool water and apply a mineral oil-free moisturizer. Both the plum and the egg white will draw out excess oils and debris from your pores, without drying out your skin. The vitamins, minerals and high antioxidant content in the plums will nourish and feed your skin the necessary nutrients it needs for healthy skin rejuvenation, fading skin discolorations and moisture-retention benefits. For maximum beauty benefits, use this plum mask 3 times a week, ideally before bed.

3. When it comes to bone health, studies found interesting positive results in post-menopausal women who regularly consumed prunes. As older women know, osteoporosis is a big concern during menopausal years, due to the body's decline of female hormones. When study participants, all post-menopausal women, were asked to consume 100 grams of dried plums daily, the researchers found a marked improvement in bone formation markers after only 3 months. Researchers are still looking as to all the reasons why this is, but some of them include the fact that plums and prunes are loaded with antioxidant properties, and in fact, contain over twice the level of antioxidants found in blueberries or raisins. And, prunes (dried plums) seem to have an even higher antioxidant quotient than fresh plums do, making them an

important dietary addition in the prevention of free radical damage, oxidative stress and cellular inflammation to the body. Additionally, prunes contain high amounts of potassium and boron, two very important minerals needed by the body for the growth and maintenance of bone density. How many prunes equal 100 grams? 10-12 prunes a day.

4. If you're looking to lower your levels of bad cholesterol (LDL), both plums and prunes offer cholesterol-reducing benefits. For starters, the insoluble fiber found in plums and prunes inhibits the enzyme activity responsible for cholesterol production in the liver, thus helping to lower blood cholesterol levels. Secondly, the soluble fiber found in plums and prunes helps to lower cholesterol by binding itself to bile acids (compounds produced by the body to digest fats), thus purging the bile acids from the body through bowel movements. What happens in the body when bile acids are excreted is that the body is stimulated to produce more bile acids, which utilizes any stored cholesterol during manufacturing, thus lowering the body's level of cholesterol in the process.

5. A daily glass of unsweetened prune juice can help reduce the incidence of herpes simplex I and II outbreaks, as well as reduce the duration time and severity of symptoms. Credit goes to the anti-viral and anti-herpes

properties of the caffeic acid and tannins found in prune juice, which help by neutralizing and preventing multiplication of the virus. If you have a herpes outbreak, drink 2 glasses of unsweetened prune juice a day until symptoms subside. And, for the prevention of outbreaks, drink one glass daily, and in both cases, it's best to drink on an empty stomach.

Pomegranates:

Unlike most other fruits and vegetables, pomegranates do not continue to ripen once picked. They are quite hardy fruits, and will keep on your kitchen counter at room temperature for up to a month, as long as they have not been cut open. Once cut open, store any remaining fruit and seeds in a sealable plastic container and consume within 3 days. To keep pomegranates longer, you can also store them uncut in a plastic bag in the fridge for up to 2 months.

1. A staple ingredient in Ayurvedic medicine, pomegranate seeds have long been used for the removal of intestinal parasites, including tapeworm, pinworm and roundworm. Many people suffer from intestinal parasites, and don't even know it. Intestinal parasites can

be picked-up through unsafe meat preparation, poor hygiene and sanitation practices, travel abroad, as well as coming in contact with them incidentally by touching or ingesting infected feces in food, water or soil. Symptoms include un-resolving gas, bloating, fatigue, vomiting, diarrhea, stomach pain and itching around the rectum. Eating pomegranate seeds daily helps to expel parasites and prevent re-infestation. The alkaloids in pomegranate seeds sedate the parasites, making them lost their grip on the intestinal walls, making them easier to expel, as well as create an environment that is unfriendly for parasites to return.

2. Did you know that pomegranates contain 3 times as many antioxidants as red wine or green tea, and in fact, contain more antioxidants than any other natural food source. For this reason, adding pomegranates to your anti-aging diet will help to protect damage to your DNA, protect your heart, lungs, liver and other vital organs from oxidative stress and cellular inflammation, thereby reducing your risk of cancer, premature aging, and age-related conditions such as Alzheimer's disease, osteoporosis, heart attack, diabetes and stroke. Pomegranate's unique antioxidants not only breakup dangerous plaque build-up from your arteries, it also helps to breakup dangerous plaque buildup from your teeth, helping to reduce your risk of not only heart

disease and heart attack, but also bad breath, gingivitis and other teeth and gum diseases. And, if that weren't enough, both the pulp and seeds of pomegranates have superior anti-inflammatory properties, helping to fend off the pain, inflammation and stiffness associated with conditions such as arthritis, gout and rheumatism. To get all these amazing anti-aging health benefits, add pomegranate into your diet 3 times a week, eating both the pulp and seeds. You can eat the fruit alone, mixed in a smoothie, or tossed in a fruit or vegetable salad.

3. Whether you mash it on your face, ingest it, or better yet do both, pomegranate does some amazing things for your skin. The ellagic acid found in pomegranate seeds offers natural protection to your skin against the ravages of the sun, including sunburn, sun-related wrinkles, skin discoloration, and even helping to inhibit the growth of skin tumors. Pomegranate encourages cell rejuvenation to both topical and deep layers of the skin, aiding in skin tissue repair and wound healing. Adding to these benefits, pomegranate stimulates both collagen, and elastin production, helping to keep the skin plump, moist and firm. The unique omega-5 fatty acids in the fruits work to hydrate and prevent moisture loss in the skin, while at the same time combating acne and healing facial irritations and scarring related to severe breakouts. To get these skin saving

benefits, consume pomegranate regularly (both the pulp and seeds), and once or twice a week mash a fresh pomegranate, seeds and all, across freshly washed skin and let stand for 30 minutes before rinsing off with cool water.

4. In addition to pomegranate's incredible antioxidant quotient, studies in 1996 discovered that pomegranate extract was able to destroy several viruses practically on contact. I've not been able to find exactly which viruses those were, but suffice it to say, this is huge news in protecting your body naturally from foreign invaders such as viral stomach flu, and other viral infections. And of course, pharmaceutical companies prefer to hide such information from the public, instead trying to replicate these results in the laboratory and selling it to the public as a drug. In other countries where holistic therapies are much more accepted by their governments, such as India, China, Japan and New Zealand, just to name a few, pomegranate is recommended for the prevention and treatment of viral and bacterial illnesses, in the form of fresh fruit, dried seeds, extract and powders.

5. To remedy the symptoms of a sore throat, such as tightness, pain, and a raw, scratchiness, try out this do-it-yourself pomegranate elixir. First, smash up 2 pomegranates into small pieces, being sure

to save the outside bark, pulp and seeds. Smashing them inside a large Ziploc baggie helps to contain all the parts. Place all the pomegranate pieces into a saucepan with 2 cups of filtered water, and bring to a boil. Immediately reduce heat, and simmer until liquid reduces to half the amount. Remove from heat and strain. Take 1-2 tablespoons of this pomegranate elixir every few hours for quick relief from sore throat symptoms, including those caused by colds and flu's. The pomegranate's antiseptic properties help to kill off bacteria, while the antioxidant and anti-inflammatory properties will help calm irritated throat tissues and swelling, and the phytonutrients will to work to speed healing. If needed, you can make in larger batches and keep in the fridge for a week at a time. If you wish to keep it fresh longer, you can add some brandy or vodka to it, but then do not give to children. Alcohol-infused pomegranate elixir should last a couple months when kept in a tightly sealed container in the fridge.

Potatoes:

If you ask most kids what their favorite vegetable is, they'd probably say potatoes. If you ask adults what their favorite vegetable is, they might not say potatoes, but we sure do eat an enormous amount of them. Baked, fried, mashed, boiled, and every way in-between, potatoes are a staple item in grocery stores, restaurants and people's homes. You might not expect potatoes to have a lot of nutrients in them, but in truth, they are loaded with antioxidants, vitamins, minerals, flavonoids and even fiber. Amazingly, even though potatoes are heavy in weight, they are made up of 80% water. If you're going to use your potatoes within a few days, they'll keep on your kitchen counter, as long as they're kept out of direct light. Otherwise, the best place to store your spuds is in a cool, dark location such as a pantry, closet, cabinet or garage (as long as it doesn't get too hot). Additionally, the vented plastic bag that you purchase potatoes in is the best place to keep them in as you use them up. And, never store onions and potatoes near each other.

1. To help improve conditions such as acne, skin rashes, dermatitis, eczema and psoriasis, raw potato slices are an amazing skin healer. Some of raw potatoes active ingredients include phosphorus, sulphur, chlorine and potassium. All of these are

minerals crucial to the health and condition of our skin. Additionally, the high vitamin C content in raw potatoes, as well as their live enzymes, combine together to become an ideal natural food for skin. Raw potato juice is alkaline in nature and is a natural antiseptic. To use raw potatoes for any of these skin conditions, after first washing face and allowing to air dry, run a couple slices of raw potatoes across the affected areas of skin you wish to heal. Allow the potato juice to dry on skin, and leave on for 1 hour before rinsing off with cool water. The raw potato juice will unclog and pull out excess oil and debris from your pores, tighten skin, kill off bacteria, help bring skin into pH balance, soothe inflammation and encourage new healthy skin cell rejuvenation. For severe skin cases, you can use this remedy daily until condition improves, then reduce it down to several times a week for healthy skin maintenance.

2. If you regularly suffer from digestive problems, stubborn weight gain that you just can't lose, and chronic fatigue, you might be surprised to learn that drinking fresh potato juice daily is an effective way to purge toxins from your entire gastrointestinal system, and release build-up, stored waste matter that quite often is the cause of all these symptoms. Simultaneously, the alkaline substances in the potato bind to acidic uric acid deposits in the body and

flush them out through our excretory system, helping to bring much needed relief from the painful symptoms of arthritis, gout and rheumatism. To make fresh raw potato juice, you can either use a quality juicer, or use the following recipe. In the evening before bed, wash and grate a large, organic potato and place the shavings into a tall glass of distilled water, along with a pinch of sea salt (do not ever use commercial table salt). Let potato soak overnight, and in the morning strain out the potato shavings and drink on an empty stomach within 30 minutes of waking. You can do this each morning for 2-3 weeks, for a nice complete body cleanse, and thereafter do it several days each week, to help prevent toxic build-up. You should notice a difference in your food cravings as well, because when your body is free of toxic waste, it starts to crave healthy food choices and will naturally shun fast food, alcohol and processed junk food.

3. For instances of infected sores, oozing wounds, poison ivy and boils a warm poultice of freshly grated potatoes will go to work quickly to help heal the skin condition. Raw potatoes have powerful drawing abilities, really helping to pull out pus and other infectious fluids from the affected area, while at the same time infusing the wound with the necessary nutrients and alkaloids it needs to stimulate healing and the mending of the skin tissue. To prepare,

first grate enough raw potato to cover the affected skin area. Place the grated potato in the center of a cheesecloth, handkerchief or thin cloth, fold edges to contain the potato, and heat the poultice using a low heat setting of your iron. It should only take 1 minute on each side to warm the poultice. First make sure poultice is not too hot to place against skin, then place gently over affected area. Hold or secure in place, and let sit for 30-60 minutes before removing. You can do this every 4 hours for acute conditions, or once daily for milder conditions. As always, if your wound is bleeding or otherwise unmanageable, seek medical attention.

4. For fast removal of embarrassing warts, potato peels are quite effective. Warts are an external sign of an internal potassium deficiency. The combination of alkaloids and high natural potassium content in potatoes penetrate the skin, and go to work to kill the wart at the root. While taping duct tape against your warts can work, it often takes weeks or months to see results. Instead, peel the skin off a raw potato (as thin as you can without tearing), and tape the potato-side of the peel against your wart(s) and leave in place. You want to leave the peel on for at least 8 hours a day. Within 1-2 weeks, you should notice the warts starting to shrivel and change color, and ultimately either fall off or just dissolve. This typically works for both large and

small warts, as well as wart clusters.

5. One of the quickest ways to relieve the pain, itching and swelling of hemorrhoids, is with chilled red potato. Carefully carve a piece of raw red potato to the shape of your small finger. Place your 'potato finger' in the freezer for 15 minutes to chill, then gently insert it into your rectum and leave in place for 15 minutes before removing and discarding in the toilet. The high astringent and anti-inflammatory properties in the raw, red potato will bring down swelling, pain, itching and burning within minutes. And, all those phytonutrients in the potato will absorb into the delicate tissues in and around your rectal area, helping to heal damaged tissues.

Pumpkin and Squash:

With care, you can store pumpkins and winter squash for up to 2-3 months before using, so you can make the most out of each season's harvest. For starters, only purchase pumpkins and winter squash when they are ripe. They store best in temperatures between 50 degrees and 95 degrees Fahrenheit, and should be covered with a towel at night when temperatures could produce frost or freeze. Never store pumpkins on carpet or wood surfaces, as this can soften the pumpkin ends and cause seeping.

And, another mislabeled (knowingly) food product on store shelves is canned pumpkin. This holiday favorite for baking and cooking is actually pureed squash.

1. Raw pumpkin seeds are naturally rich in the L-tryptophan, and amino acid that stimulates the production of our body's feel-good hormone serotonin. Science reveals that those who suffer from mild depression and other mood disorders, are typically highly deficient in this important hormone. Eating raw pumpkin seeds not only helps balance mood, it also helps boost mental clarity, memory recall and focus, due to the expansive amounts of brain nourishing phytonutrients, making this an ideal food to help protect against age-related mental decline. Suggested dosage for both mood and mental boost benefits is ¼ cup daily.

2. Butternut squash is ultra-beneficial for cardiac well-being. It contains high amounts of vitamin A, folate, potassium, vitamin B6, omega-3 fatty acids, beta carotene, magnesium, calcium and other minerals, all of which are absolutely essential for optimal heart health. These phytonutrients help breakup and prevent plaque build-up on artery walls, help keep blood pressure levels stable, help reduce levels of bad cholesterol (LDL) and reduce your risk of heart disease,

heart attack and stroke. Butternut squash is easy to prepare, and you can bake it and mash it up like mashed potatoes, and drizzle with some raw maple syrup (not pancake syrup), use it in casseroles or dice it up and sauté it with some walnut or olive oil in a skillet.

3. Looking to keep your face smooth, fresh and radiant during the cool, dry autumn and early winter months? Here is a pumpkin face mask recipe you can whip up in just minutes that will help keep your skin radiant during those harsh weather months. In a mixing bowl, gently whisk together 1 tablespoon of fresh pumpkin pulp (or you can substitute 1 tablespoon canned pumpkin puree) with 1 teaspoon raw honey and 1 teaspoon heavy cream. After washing face and neck, apply pumpkin mask evenly across skin areas (face, neck, décolletage) and let sit for 30 minutes before rinsing off with cool water. It's best to lay back while the mask is on your face, because as the ingredients warm against your skin, it will start to drip. Both the pumpkin and the heavy cream offer natural acids that will gently exfoliate dead skin cells and debris, while stimulating new skin cell turnover. The mega phytonutrients in the pumpkin and raw honey, infuse your skin with antiseptic, antibacterial and antioxidant benefits, that will protect your skin against harsh winds and dry, cold air, helping to prevent windburn and dry,

cracking, peeling skin that can often occur during the cold weather months.

4. For the healing of minor burns, skin rashes, scrapes and abrasions, a poultice of cold pumpkin can bring rapid relief. To start, you need to place enough raw pumpkin pulp (or use canned pumpkin puree) to cover affected skin area into the freezer for 1 hour to chill. After the hour, place the chilled pumpkin puree into the center of a piece of cheesecloth, handkerchief or other thin cloth, and fold to make a poultice pouch. Gently place onto the affected area, and hold in place against the skin for 30-60 minutes. The pumpkin will go to work to draw out any infectious fluid and debris from the area, as well as infuse it will nutrients the skin needs to heal. When the body is deficient in zinc, it delays wound healing and skin mending. Pumpkin is not only loaded with zinc, it's also rich in skin nourishing vitamin A, essential fatty acids and antioxidants which will neutralize free radical damage and inflammation that has occurred to the skin area.

5. Most dieters might be surprised to learn that winter squashes are very diet friendly. All of the winter squash varieties are very high in fiber, with acorn squash coming out on top with 9 grams of dietary fiber per single serving. Foods that are high in natural dietary fiber help keep blood sugar levels

stable and prevent overeating and food cravings for unhealthy food choices. They also fill you up faster, and keep you feeling full longer. Additionally, the carbohydrates found in winter squashes are very unique in that even though they contain starch compounds, they don't react the same way as starch from rice, noodles, breads and processed foods do. Winter squashes starch compounds actually contain antioxidant, anti-inflammatory and insulin-regulating properties, making it a better carbohydrate food choice for diabetics and dieters.

Radishes:

Radishes are pretty much available year-round, and come in a handful of varieties. The most common is the globe radish, which looks a bit like a cherry tomato. Other varieties include black radish, daikon radish, icicle radish and mammoth white radish. Typically radishes are sold in a 'bunch', still attached to its greens. Once you purchase radishes, it is best to separate the radish bulbs from the greens and store separately, otherwise the greens will absorb too much moisture and nutrients, and deteriorate the radish rather quickly. When separated, the radish bulbs will keep fresh for approximately 5 days or so, and the radish greens about 2 days. For you gardeners, radishes have natural pesticide properties, helping to fend off garden insects and critters due to their spicy, peppery oils.

1. Fresh radishes are truly a dieter's dream, in that they are proven to eliminate hardened imbedded fat from body tissues, thus helping one to shed excess weight, eliminate stored toxins and smooth out unsightly cellulite. Additionally, eating fresh radish helps the body to breakdown and digest starchy foods, such as grains, pasta, potatoes, rice and the like, making it a great addition, or at least an edible garnish, to carbohydrate-rich dishes. For a potent whole body detoxifier and weight loss aid, try this morning detox juice recipe. In a juicer, put through 3-4 carrots, 2 large radishes and ½ of a large lemon. Drink on an empty stomach within 30 minutes of waking. This is also a great morning-after drink to consume after an evening of overeating, especially during holiday season.

2. One of the best methods for naturally healing a chronic cough, inflamed sore throat, laryngitis and phlegm, is this ancient Chinese remedy using daikon radish. Just grate up several radishes, and drizzle with a small amount of raw honey. Eat a teaspoon every few hours as needed for fast relief of your symptoms. The radish-honey

combination offers potent antibacterial and antiseptic properties that will kill harmful bacteria in your throat, mouth and digestive tract, while loosening up any accompanying phlegm so it can be expelled, and soothe inflamed throat and mouth tissues. Because this remedy involved raw honey, do not give to children under the age of 2 years. An alternative recipe, is to blend or juice together 1 onion and 3 radishes, and take a teaspoon every few hours. The taste is quite strong, but this radish combination is equally as effective.

3. To prevent a morning-after hangover, or remedy one that has already hit you, here is one of the very best hangover remedies in the world of natural remedies. Peel and grate ½ cup of daikon radish into a mixing bowl, and stir in ½ tablespoon fresh squeezed lemon juice, ½ tablespoon of chia seeds, and a pinch of sea salt. Once all ingredients are mixed together, eat the entire mixture followed by a glass of water. The radish is highly detoxifying to the body, especially the liver, and aids in the rapid breakdown of the alcohol within the body. The chia seeds have high levels of omega-3 fatty acids which support cell regeneration, and, they can retain up to 24 times their weight in water. So, as the daikon radish pulls toxins from your cell tissues, the chia seeds absorb these toxins and the lemon helps flush them from your body. The sea salt replenishes

minerals that were lost due to drinking alcohol. Also remember to drink extra water throughout the day, so your body can expel the toxins that the radish hangover remedy is working hard at to remove.

4. Rubbing radish juice or grated radish on your face, is a natural skin lightener, and will help fade age spots, freckles, scars and other skin discolorations. To use, simply juice or grate several fresh radishes (any variety will work), and apply to freshly washed skin. Leave residue on for 20-30 minutes before rinsing with cool water. With regular use, you'll notice a definite brightening, whitening and clearing of your skin tone. The radish juice is also very antiseptic, and will help cleanse skin of pore-clogging oils and debris, while also shrinking the pores and tightening the skin.

5. These days, more people are turning away from chemical antiperspirants and deodorants, and turning to natural deodorant solutions instead. Most commercial antiperspirants contain dangerous aluminum compounds, which clog underarm pores and seep into the body, where they can do harm. In fact, most women with breast cancer, and most people with Alzheimer's disease have high levels of aluminum deposits in their body. And, this doesn't even include all the people who end up getting rashes and other allergic reactions to commercial

antiperspirants, due to the chemical they contain. To make your own effective natural deodorant, juice 24 large radishes (any variety), transfer into a large plastic squeeze bottle, and add in ¼ teaspoon glycerin, which is a natural preservative. To use, after bathing, give the radish mixture a shake to mix, and squeeze a dab into the palm of your hand. Rub your palms together, and apply evenly to your underarm area. If you would like to add a scent to the radish deodorant, you can add in 5 drops of essential oil of lavender, geranium or sandalwood. If you suffer from foot odor, you can also massage a couple drops of the radish deodorant into the soles of your feet, to help keep offensive food odor away.

Rhubarb:

Rhubarb is quite easy to grow, and one of my personal favorites in the garden. I have a personal taste preference for all things with a tangy, tart bite to them, and rhubarb provides just the right amount of sweet and tart in baking and cooking recipes. When purchasing rhubarb at the grocery store or farmers market, you want to choose firm, bright red stalks with no brown discolorations at the ends. If they still have their leaves attached, they should not be wilted, as this is a sign the rhubarb is past its prime. Only purchase what you'll use within a few days, but rhubarb does freeze well, so you can certainly prep and freeze them for future use. You'll ideally want to use your frozen rhubarb within 3 months. To store fresh rhubarb, trim off any leaves, and cut off the ends and any areas of discoloration. Wash, and wrap loosely in some paper towels before storing in a crisper drawer in the fridge. Use within 2-3 days. It's also worth noting, that rhubarb is one of those few very acidic vegetables, and should be avoided by those suffering from arthritis, gout and rheumatism, as it could aggravate symptoms.

1. While no claims are being made, rhubarb has been long used in anti-cancer diets. Two of the compounds found in rhubarb that give it its laxative properties, rhein and emodin, have been shown in scientific studies to also have anti-tumor value. Study results were published in the medical publications Pharmacology and Journal of Ethnopharmacology, outlining the study results, of which Ehrlich and breast tumors were able to be blocked by 75%, and malignant melanoma tumors were able to be blocked by 76%. One of the reasons behind these positive anti-tumor results is the ability of these two rhubarb compounds to inhibit the uptake of glucose in tumor cells. Cancer cells need sugar to feed on and grow, and when their 'food supply' is cut-off, it results

in cancer cell death. If you'd like to add rhubarb as an anti-cancer dietary addition to your diet, in addition to cutting out as much sugar in your diet as possible, the suggested consumption dose for rhubarb is ½ cup of fresh juiced rhubarb or 2 cups of rhubarb tea daily. To make rhubarb tea, add 2 cups of finely chopped rhubarb stalks to 1 quart of boiling water, cover pot and simmer for 1 hour. Let stand for 5 minutes, strain, and drink 1 cup 2-3 times a day.

2. Summertime means lots of outdoor activities. And, if you spend a lot of time hiking through dense wooded areas or fields, it means you have an increased risk of picking-up a case of painful poison ivy or poison oak. The rash, blisters, and itching that accompany these conditions is very unpleasant. Fortunately, rhubarb is widely available in the summer months (conveniently so by Mother Nature's design), and it is quite effective at bringing rapid relief to all of your uncomfortable symptoms. Simply boil down some chopped rhubarb in plain water, and gently swab the affected skin areas with the rhubarb water using cotton balls, and allow residue to air dry on skin. Apply every few hours, and be sure to discard the cotton balls after each use to avoid recontamination. You'll notice relief from itching within about 15 minutes, and if you commit to apply the rhubarb water every few hours, you should have

significant, if not complete healing within 2 days.

3. For rapid relief from heartburn and indigestion, do what the Native Americans do, and eat a stalk of well-chilled rhubarb. Eating a stalk of raw rhubarb has a calming effect on the stomach, and helps to neutralize excessive stomach acid, acting as a natural antacid. For antacid benefits, you must eat the rhubarb raw, as it doesn't seem to have the same effect once cooked. Additionally, eating some raw rhubarb after a meal also aids in regulating your digestive system, helping to prevent both constipation and diarrhea, making it a perfect edible garnish to include with your meal.

4. For gardeners, rhubarb leaves make an excellent insecticide against unwanted leaf-eating garden insects. In a large saucepan, shred up a few pounds of rhubarb leaves into a quart of water, and cook at a slow boil for 15 minutes. Remove from heat and allow mixture to cool. Strain into a plastic spray bottle, and add in a couple squirts of liquid dishwashing detergent and shake to mix. Spray your garden plants once a week with the rhubarb garden mixture, to help prevent insects from dining on your garden plants.

5. For those with natural blond or light brown hair, who find that their color is fading and dull due to age, rhubarb makes a powerful,

natural hair dye that can bring color and brightness back to your lackluster locks. To make, finely dice ½ cup of fresh rhubarb root and add it to a saucepan (glass or stainless steel only) filled with 1 quart distilled water (ONLY use distilled water). Bring to a boil, reduce heat and simmer covered for 20 minutes. Do not lift lid during simmering time. Remove from heat, and let mixture steep overnight. The next day, strain out the rhubarb pieces and transfer liquid into a small pitcher or measuring cup. To use, wash hair as usual, then hanging your head over a large pot or bowl to catch the fluid, pour the rhubarb rinse through your hair and run your fingers or a wide-toothed comb through to evenly distribute the rinse. Repeat 3 times with the captured rhubarb liquid, re-combing after each rinse. Allow hair to air dry without any additional rinsing. You'll notice an immediate lightened and brightened color to your hair, without the use of any harsh chemicals.

Spinach:

You'd be hard-pressed to find a vegetable that has a higher nutrient content than spinach. Spinach is loaded with vitamins K, A, C and even B vitamins. It's a rich source of iron, calcium, magnesium and other vital minerals. And, then there is the mass-amounts of flavonoids and carotenoids found in spinach, giving it incredible antioxidant properties. It even contains healthy omega-3 fatty acids. When purchasing fresh spinach, you want to select bright, crisp bunches, and avoid limp and lifeless looking ones. Never wash spinach until you're ready to use it, and when storing spinach, it will stay fresh for up to 5 days when wrapped loosely in paper towels and kept in the crisper drawer in the fridge. And, the best way to retain all these amazing nutrients in spinach is to eat it raw, steamed or quick-boiled (1 minute or less). Additionally, spinach is another one of those vegetables that you really want to only buy organic. Pesticide and herbicide residues cling easily to spinach's leaves, and washing will never remove them all, which ultimately means you'll be ingesting these leftover chemical residues.

1. For those aged 40 and over, regularly eating spinach will help aid in maintaining healthy, strong bones throughout your latter years. A single serving (1 cup) of quick-boiled spinach yields 1000% of your daily

recommended vitamin K, a vitamin crucial to good bone health. Spinach not only provides ample amounts of calcium and magnesium, the vitamin K content in spinach helps to 'lock in' the calcium and magnesium to the bone, exactly where it is needed. Additionally, vitamin K1 helps prevent the breakdown of bone density, while vitamin K2 stimulates new bone growth. Spinach is easily prepared in so many ways, making it easy to fit this healthy vegetable into your daily diet. You can juice it, use it in salads, for sandwich wraps, stir-fry's, sautéed with some raw walnuts and so much more.

2. If you're living with fatigue, cooked spinach is a natural energizing vegetable that can help you overcome your debilitating symptoms. I emphasize cooked (steamed, boiled, sautéed, etc.), because spinach is classified as a goitrogen, which means it suppresses thyroid function when eaten in its raw state. Cooking spinach disables the enzymes that are responsible for impairing healthy thyroid function. Therefore, you can enjoy the natural energy boost without further aggravating your thyroid symptoms. The energy boost you get from consuming cooked spinach comes from its rich stores of iron, folate, vitamin C, magnesium and B vitamins, as well as its anti-inflammatory flavonoid compounds. All these phytonutrients strengthen the blood as well

as the function of the adrenal glands, which is a major cause of chronic fatigue in many people today (referring to adrenal exhaustion). So, if you regularly struggle with fatigue, start adding some cooked spinach to your diet at least 3-4 times a week.

3. To help clear up stubborn acne, skin rashes, dermatitis and other skin imbalances, using fresh spinach both internally and externally can help clear up even the most stubborn of cases within 1-2 weeks. The all-star lineup of phytonutrients found in spinach, are all incredibly nourishing and balancing to skin. Used topically, spinach juice helps to draw out pore-clogging oils and debris, while stimulating new skin cell turnover. Used internally, spinach helps flush accumulated acidic waste from cell tissues (a major contributing factor to skin disorders), balancing your body's pH levels. To make a healthy spinach juice you can drink daily, here is a good recipe that you can adjust to taste preference. In a blender or juicer, combine ½ of a fresh bundle of spinach, 2 ripe tomatoes and 1 large cucumber (peeled), and blend until smooth. Transfer into a serving glass, and drink. You can also add in a splash of hot sauce or black pepper to kick-it up a bit. If you have a juicer, you can try combining spinach with carrots, beets, collard greens, apples and pears. All of which, are also very nourishing for the

skin. To use spinach topically, just blend or juice 1 large bunch of spinach, and saturate a cotton ball with the juice and apply to freshly washed skin. Allow to sit for 15-30 minutes, before rinsing with cool water. Store the remaining spinach juice in a closed container, and store in the fridge. Leftover juice can be used within 5 days. For severe skin cases, use this remedy daily for 2 weeks, then 2-3 times a week for maintenance. For milder cases, use 1-2 times a week.

4. An effective and safe natural diuretic recipe that will help flush out stored toxic fluids from the body, as well as aid in healing the symptoms of UTI (urinary tract infection) and cystitis, is a simple juice combination of fresh spinach and coconut water. The combination of nitrates and potassium help to unlock and release trapped fluids, and can even help increase urine output that may be otherwise restricted due to medication or dehydration. To make this easy recipe, just combine 1 can of coconut water (do not use coconut milk or cream), with ½ bunch of fresh spinach in a blender, and blend until smooth. If you need a little flavor enhancer, you can add in some freshly squeezed lime juice from ½ of a large, ripe lime. You can drink this at any time throughout the day, but drinking it first thing in the morning on an empty stomach is preferred.

5. To help calm a dry, scratchy cough, as well as soothe inflamed throat and lung tissues, here is an effective spinach remedy you can whip up in minutes. In a blender, combine ½ bunch of fresh spinach with 1 tablespoon of raw honey, and blend until smooth. Transfer into a small saucepan, and gently warm. Remove from heat and take 1 tablespoon of the mixture every couple hours, for rapid relief of symptoms. The combination of strong anti-inflammatory and antioxidant properties in both the spinach and honey quickly go to work to reduce swelling, irritation and coughing. Do not give to children under 2 years of age, due to the honey content.

Tomatoes:

While potatoes may be a top ranking vegetable, at least here in the United States, tomatoes probably rank up there as one of the top ranking fruits consumed in the United States. And, in a surprising bit of trivia, in 1893 the Supreme Court ruled to reclassify tomatoes as an official vegetable, even though botanically speaking, they will never be a vegetable. I have no clue as to how or why tomatoes made their way into the Supreme Court, or who would have even benefitted from the resulting decision. Perhaps lobbyists were already around back then. As for storing tomatoes, fresh picked tomatoes, or those purchased from a farmers market store best at room temperature for up to a week, out of direct sunlight. Ideally, they should be placed in a large, shallow bowl, lined with a couple paper towels. Unfortunately, tomatoes purchased at a grocery store have already been subjected to refrigeration, and will not keep well unrefrigerated at home, even though that's how they store best. If you purchase tomatoes that are encased in a plastic wrap, immediately remove the plastic when you get home, to allow the tomatoes to 'breathe', and prevent premature deterioration.

1. If a day out in the sun has left you with areas of sunburn, tomatoes can quickly soothe the pain and tightness of the burn, while at the same time going to work to infuse the affected areas with skin healing properties. As soon as you can, puree 2 parts ripe tomatoes to 1 part buttermilk, using enough ingredients to cover affected sunburned skin area. Once you have the tomato-buttermilk mixture blended, put it in the freezer for 30 minutes to chill before using. After the mixture is well chilled, but not frozen, gently apply it to affected areas, and let it sit for at least 30 minutes before gently rinsing off with cool-cold water. The sooner you can apply this remedy, and the longer you let it stay on the skin, especially the first application, the more significant will be

relief and healing to the area. The mixture will bring almost instant pain relief, while going to work to correct the skin's pH balance, which is has been damaged from the sunburn. The tomatoes high vitamin C content, which is a potent antioxidant, will neutralize the free radical damage caused by the excessive sun exposure, and the high amounts of vitamin A will stimulate the growth of new, healthy skin cells to replace the sun-damaged one. Never, ever apply butter, baby oil, petroleum jelly or other oil-based product to a burn, as these substances will clog pores and create a skin barrier that prevents heat from escaping from the skin, thus causing further damage to the skin.

2. To combat the effects of aging as well as sun-damage to skin, tomatoes are highly effective at reversing the physical effects of both. Tomatoes are rich in the nutrient lycopene, a carotenoid that neutralizes free radicals that can accelerate aging of the skin, resulting in fine lines, wrinkles, sagging and dry, crepey, loose skin. Lycopene also gives the skin an element of protection against photo-damage (sun damage), thus helping to minimize the risk of skin discoloration, textural changes and skin cancer, that might be caused by excessive sun exposure. In addition to eating lots of fresh, organic tomatoes in your diet, you can also use tomatoes topically for even better results. Studies also show that the nutrient lycopene

is better absorbed by the body when combined with a healthy oil, so when eating, drizzle your tomatoes with some extra-virgin olive oil. And, when using topically, your added oil can be olive oil, coconut oil or even raw honey. A simple skin rejuvenating facial mask recipe can be made by combining 1 large, ripe tomato, 1 teaspoon honey and 1 teaspoon plain yogurt in a blender, and puree until smooth. Apply to freshly washed skin areas (face, neck, décolletage) and let sit for 30 minutes before rinsing with cool water. Using this mask 3 times a week will bring amazing transformational results to age and sun-damaged skin, and if you spend a lot of time outdoors during the summer months, use this mask as often as you can for prevention measures.

3. An unbelievably easy way to use fresh tomato slices, is for the healing of skin wounds, such as abrasions, cuts, rashes, and even oozing sores. Simply tape a thin slice of tomato large enough to cover affected area with medical tape or a bandage, and change every few hours for rapid healing of the skin condition. Repeat as needed until condition resolves. Tomatoes are loaded with ascorbic acid, a necessary nutrient required by the body for wound healing, wound closure, infection prevention and healthy new skin formation. And, tomatoes rich vitamin A content helps to minimize

scarring and renew damaged skin.

4. For those with fatigue and lethargy, you may be suffering from low iron, as is the case with anemia. Tomatoes are not only rich in iron, but the iron from tomatoes is readily absorbed into the stomach and intestines and is completely assimilated into the body. Drinking fresh tomato juice (not canned or bottled) is a perfect pick-me drink for those suffering from low iron counts, low energy and brain fog, making it a much healthier and more effective beverage choice vs. chemical and sugar-laden 'energy drinks'. You don't even need a juicer. Simply through 4-5 large, ripe tomatoes into a blender with some salt and pepper, or a splash of lemon juice and hot sauces and puree until smooth.

5. To remedy the pain and unsightliness of external or internal mouth sores, including canker sores, here is a tomato recipe that will help bring rapid healing as well as much needed pain relief. In a blender, puree together 2 ripe tomatoes with 2 fresh basil leaves (only use fresh ingredients) until smooth and transfer into a small dish. To use, first rinse mouth out with warm water, to remove any surface debris. Next, dab on the tomato-basil mixture to mouth sores, and let sit as long as possibly before rinsing. The tomato contains ascorbic acid, which stimulates wound healing and reduces

outbreak time. Both the tomato and basil also contain antiseptic properties to help kill off harmful mouth bacteria. And, the basil also contains potent antiviral properties, helping to heal sores that may be due to the herpes virus. Use as often as needed until condition improves.

Tropical Fruits:

Tropical fruits are cultivated in countries and states with warm climates, and the only characteristic all tropical fruit varieties share, is their intolerance to frost and freezing temperatures. Thankfully, due to modern shipping methods, we can enjoy tropical fruits in most regions of the world. While there is a vast array of tropical fruits to choose from, we'll just be covering a few of the most common, such as papaya, mango, pineapple and guava. When purchasing these fruits, they should all feel firm to the touch, and slightly heavy. Avoid buying specimens with tears, bruising, soft spots, or wrinkly, weathered skin exteriors. All of these fruits store well at room temperature when they are still unripe, and then should be transferred to the fridge once they become ripened.

1. Both papaya and pineapple are very useful in getting rid of warts and corns in short

order. In both cases, either the fruit or the peel can be used however, the peel yields faster and better results, and seems to be where most of the wart and corn-dissolving properties tend to be. Step one is to first soak foot (or feet, hand, hands) in a tub of hot water for 10 minutes. Remove and allow skin to air dry. Next, cut a piece of your choice of papaya or pineapple peel large enough to cover the wart or corn, place it over the affected area, and secure it tightly in place with some wide medical tape or bandage. You want to always be sure to place the inside of the cut peel against the wart or corn. If using on feet, you can easily slip on a pair of socks over your secured bandage. Leave on day and night, changing fresh peel and bandage twice a day. This method will shrivel up and dissolve warts and corns quickly, and even stubborn cases will respond, though they might take a little longer.

2. Fresh pineapple and fresh pineapple juice are both very detoxifying to the body, and supportive to digestive health. For starters, pineapples are loaded with an enzyme called bromelain, which not only breaks down protein molecules in the foods we eat, it also is a natural anti-inflammatory, so it soothes inflamed throat, stomach and intestinal tissues. This means that you'll be better able to digest and assimilate food, and reduce your risk of heartburn, excess gas and

bloating. The fiber, diuretic and mineral properties of pineapple give it its ability to flush out stored toxic waste from cell tissues, allowing them to be expelled from the body. Trapped toxic waste leads to skin disruptions, weight gain, digestive disturbances and eventually on to other more serious health conditions. Eating canned pineapple or canned and bottle pineapple juice does NOT offer the same benefits, as the live enzymes and nutrients have been destroyed during the pasteurization and other processing of the final end product. In other words, only fresh pineapple with do.

3. Immature guavas (un-ripened) are highly astringent, and are very beneficial in tightening and toning loose, sagging, crepey skin on the neck, otherwise known as 'turkey neck'. For a do-it-yourself skin-tightening recipe, combine 1 diced un-ripened guava, along with all its leaves into a blender, along with a splash of coconut milk and puree until smooth. Apply to freshly washed skin on the neck and décolletage area, then lay back and let sit on skin for 30-60 minutes before rinsing off with cool water. For even more skin toning benefits, reserve a piece of cut guava, and after rinsing off the guava-coconut mask, rub the piece of cut guava across the neck and décolletage and let the residue stay on overnight before rinsing off in the morning. This will allow all those rich antioxidants

and skin-rejuvenating nutrients in the guava to deeply penetrate your skin, further speeding up your skin toning and tightening results.

4. If you're a chronic dieter, you've probably heard about the positive effects mango has for weight loss. And, I personally suspect that eating the raw fruit may yield better results over taking mango in supplement form. For starters, mango is rich in natural dietary fiber, which means that eating it will help you become full faster, and stay full longer. Plus, dietary fiber naturally scrubs your intestinal tract of accumulated toxic waste matter, which left unchecked can lead to stubborn weight gain that won't come off. Next, mango is absolutely loaded with healthy weight supporting nutrients, helping to fend off unhealthy food cravings and overeating. When we are stuck in a cycle of overeating, it's not because we haven't consumed enough volume of food, it's because we haven't consumed enough of the necessary nutrients are body requires, such as vitamins, minerals and amino acids. Therefore, the body triggers our hunger signal prematurely in a desperate attempt to acquire these necessary nutrients. Consuming fresh mango will help supply your body with these necessary nutrients, naturally squashing any premature hunger signals. How much should you eat to support weight loss? Eating 1-2 fresh

mangos as your breakfast, along with some herbal or green tea in the morning, will support healthy and sustaining weight loss.

5. Ladies, if you're looking to firm and increase your bust-line naturally, without dangerous surgery, here is an ancient recipe that's been used successfully to tone and enlarge women's breasts in Asian countries as well as India. Dice up 1-2 un-ripened, green papayas, and add them to a large saucepan with 2 cups of apple cider vinegar with the 'mother' enzyme and 1 cup of distilled water. Bring to a rolling boil, then reduce heat, cover and simmer on low heat for 1 hour. Remove from heat, and let steep for an additional 15 minutes. Using a small strainer, strain the mixture into a sealable jar or other container and store in fridge. Each day, take 1 tablespoon 5-6 times during your waking hours. The mixture can be quite tart and pungent, and for this reason it may be easier to consume with a small amount of food, preferably some fresh fruit or vegetables. No claims are being made, but women are reported to start noticing results within the first 10-30 days, and with continued use the results remain.

ADDITIONAL BOOKS BY AUTHOR:

- Easy Vegetarian Cooking: 100 – 5 Ingredients or Less, Easy and Delicious Vegetarian Recipes

- Easy Vegetarian Cooking: 75 Delicious Vegetarian Casserole Recipes

- Easy Vegetarian Cooking: 75 Delicious Vegetarian Soup and Stew Recipes

- Natural Foods: 100 – 5 Ingredients or Less, Raw Food Recipes for Every Meal Occasion

- The Veggie Goddess Vegetarian Cookbook Collection: Volumes 1-4

- Easy Vegan Cooking: 100 Easy & Delicious Vegan Recipes

- Vegan Cooking: 50 Vegan Dessert Recipes

- Holiday Vegan Recipes: Holiday Menu Planning for Halloween through New Years

- The Veggie Goddess Vegan Cookbooks Collection: Volumes 1-3

ABOUT THE AUTHOR

Gina 'The Veggie Goddess' Matthews, resides in sunny Phoenix, Arizona, and has been a lover of animals, nature, gardening and vegetarian and vegan cuisine since childhood. 'The Veggie Goddess' strongly encourages home gardening, supporting your local farmers and organic food co-ops, protecting animal rights, and preserving the well-being of Mother Earth.

www.ingramcontent.com/pod-product-compliance
Lightning Source LLC
Chambersburg PA
CBHW070009300526
45794CB00001B/256